Preterm
Birth

Preterm birth is a significant cause of neonatal mortality and morbidity, with a devastating impact on families. This essential guide introduces the knowledge that midwives require for practice, drawing together the most up-to-date research and identifying care pathways.

Preterm Birth: A Handbook for Midwives presents the latest evidence, discussing the causes and consequences of preterm birth. It describes what preterm birth is, explores the risk factors and causes, explains monitoring methods and presents interventions for reducing the risk of preterm birth itself as well as interventions for managing its consequences. Women's voices are heard throughout as they describe their experiences in their own words, and each substantive chapter includes recommendations for practice.

Compact and accessible, this practical guide is an indispensable handbook, enabling students and qualified midwives to care confidently for women at risk of preterm birth.

Naomi Carlisle is a midwifery lecturer at King's College London, UK. She recently defended her PhD thesis regarding implementation of the preterm birth pathway in England, and has previously worked clinically in the Preterm Birth Surveillance Clinic at St Thomas' Hospital, London, UK.

Jenny Carter is a midwife and Senior Research Fellow at King's College London and the Tommy's National Centre for Preterm Birth Research. Her PhD thesis focused on risk assessment in threatened preterm labour and development of the QUiPP app. She is a founder member of the UK Preterm Clinical Network, and she also works clinically in the Preterm Surveillance Clinic at St Thomas' Hospital.

This must-read handbook is a comprehensive, factual and informative handbook, and an excellent resource for midwives and students. The chapters are full of essential knowledge, that assists the reader in understanding the risks, causes, prediction markers and interventions associated with preterm birth and the specialist care required.

Professor Jacqueline Dunkley-Bent OBE
Chief Midwife, International Confederation of Midwives (ICM)

Preterm birth is complex, and strategies to tackle this enormous problem are rapidly evolving. This is an excellent resource, written by clinicians with immense experience, clearly written and easy to understand, covering both essential and contemporary knowledge in the subject. I can highly recommend it.

Professor Andrew Shennan OBE
International Federation of Gynecology and Obstetrics (FIGO)
Preterm Birth Committee Chair (2021–2023)

A fantastic resource for midwives and student midwives wishing to gain a greater insight into all aspects of preterm birth. This book is comprehensive and highly informative. A must read for clinical midwives looking to improve preterm birth services.

Gemma Miller
Preterm birth specialist midwives NHS Network Chair

Preterm
Birth

A Handbook for Midwives

Naomi Carlisle and Jenny Carter

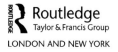

Routledge
Taylor & Francis Group

LONDON AND NEW YORK

Designed cover image: Getty image number 965683524

First published 2025
by Routledge
4 Park Square, Milton Park, Abingdon, Oxon OX14 4RN

and by Routledge
605 Third Avenue, New York, NY 10158

Routledge is an imprint of the Taylor & Francis Group, an informa business

British Library Cataloguing-in-Publication Data
A catalogue record for this book is available from the British Library

ISBN: 978-1-032-46194-6 (hbk)
ISBN: 978-1-032-46193-9 (pbk)
ISBN: 978-1-003-38050-4 (ebk)

DOI: 10.4324/9781003380504

Typeset Helvetica
by KnowledgeWorks Global Ltd.

We would like to dedicate this book to all the women and their families who have experienced preterm birth and mid-trimester loss.

Contents

Figures

Tables

Foreword

I am honoured to provide a foreword for this handbook for midwives written by midwives. The aim of this handbook is to assist midwives in developing a knowledge and understanding about preterm birth and to build confidence in providing optimal care for women at risk.

Why is this such an important topic? Preterm birth comprises around 8% of births in England and Wales, and prematurity is the most significant cause of mortality in children under five and is associated with significant morbidity in surviving infants. Furthermore, the rates of preterm birth have not decreased. The latest 2023 data shows that the number of babies born preterm is increasing in the UK from 7.4% in 2020 to 7.6% in 2021. Babies from the black ethnic group have had the highest proportion of preterm births since data collection began in 2007. In 2021, 8.7% of live births in the black ethnic group were preterm births, and the biggest percentage increase in preterm live births was in the Asian ethnic group, from 7.5% to 8.1%.

Globally one in ten babies are born preterm according to World Health Organization in 2023, and no region of the world has significantly reduced rates of preterm births over the last decade in all parts of the world.

Reducing variations in quality of care is critical if the women who are at the greatest risk are to receive the care they need. But the task for the future for all of us is to focus on prevention and this will need us to think outside the box and look at the context of women's lives and the environment that we live in.

Professor Jane Sandall, CBE, FMedSci
Professor of Social Science and Women's Health at
King's College London

Preface

Being a midwife is a vocation that brings joy and responsibility, helping women through arguably the most important transition of their lives. While the role of a midwife requires them to be experts in physiological pregnancy and birth, it also requires them to identify when things deviate and to know when to seek medical advice. Midwives also care for women with complicated pregnancies and births as part of the multi-disciplinary team.

Preterm birth is a major issue, affecting many women and their families, which in recent years has gained more recognition. There are now focused national drives to reduce the preterm birth rate, and specialist preterm birth midwife roles are now established in many hospitals. Despite this, there is little information written specifically for midwives. As midwives ourselves, with many years of experience caring for women at risk of preterm birth, and in research investigating how to predict and prevent it, we decided to fill this gap. We hope this book will aid midwives, not just those working in this specialist area but also other students and midwives who would like to know more.

Having said that, please remember to always refer to your current local guidelines; the information in this book is based on our understanding at the time of writing, so new evidence and guidance may be available.

NC & JC

Acknowledgements

We would like to thank all the women who have allowed us to share their, sometimes precarious, journeys into motherhood. We have learnt so much from them and their experiences. We would also like to thank those who have contributed to our Patient and Public Involvement and Engagement activities and given advice not just on our research studies but also on our plans for this book. We have been privileged to work with some of the most wonderful, inspiring and decent colleagues – midwives, doctors and scientists – and we are particularly grateful to those who took some time to review individual chapters of this book and provided comments, corrections and ideas for improvement. These include Karen Coombes, Libby Edwards, Gemma Miller, Sam Pérez Amack, Vicky Robinson, Kate Shove, Lisa Story, Dede Thorpe and Ellie Watson. We would also like to thank Sergio Silverio, for his formatting ideas used in the Appendix. And finally, a very big thank you to Gemma Baxter, the artist who made the lovely illustrations for Figures 2.1, 3.2, 5.1 and 8.1.

NC & JC

Acronyms and abbreviations

ADU	Antenatal Day Assessment Unit
BMI	body mass index
CL	cervical length
FDCS	full dilatation caesarean section
fFN	fetal fibronectin
FIGO	International Federation of Gynecology and Obstetrics
ICM	International Confederation of Midwives
IMD	Index of Multiple Deprivation
IUT	*in utero* transfer
MHRA	Medicines and Healthcare Products Regulatory Agency
NICE	National Institute for Health and Care Excellence
NIHR	National Institute for Health Research
NNU	neonatal unit
PCN	Preterm Clinical Network (Database)
PPIE	Patient and Public Involvement and Engagement
PPROM	prelabour preterm ruptured membranes
PTB	preterm birth
PTL	preterm labour
qfFN	quantitative fetal fibronectin
RCM	Royal College of Midwives
RCOG	Royal College of Obstetricians and Gynaecologists
REC	Research Ethics Committee
sPTB	spontaneous preterm birth
TPTL	threatened preterm labour
TVS	transvaginal scan
TVS CL	transvaginal ultrasound scan measurement of cervical length
UKPCN	UK Preterm Clinical Network
UTI	urinary tract infection

Chapter 1
Why midwives need to know about preterm birth

Introduction

This book is a handbook for midwives about spontaneous preterm birth. Medically indicated (iatrogenic) preterm births, for example, for preeclampsia or suspected fetal growth restriction, account for around a third (Goldenberg *et al.*, 2008) but are not within the scope of this book. While a growing number of midwives specialise in preterm birth and perhaps even work in specialist clinics, many others have limited knowledge in this area (Carlisle *et al.*, 2024). This is despite the fact that all midwives, wherever they work, will regularly encounter women who are at risk. Since the publication of the second version of the *Saving Babies Lives Care Bundle*, with the new fifth element (NHS England, 2019), and the later version 3 (NHS England, 2023), all midwives undertaking booking appointments in England need to assess every woman for her risk of preterm birth and refer her appropriately (Carlisle *et al.*, 2024). The aim of this handbook is to assist midwives in developing a knowledge and understanding about preterm birth and to build confidence in providing optimal care for woman at risk.

This handbook covers everything a midwife needs to know, including: why it happens (Chapter 2: Causes of spontaneous preterm birth); which women are more likely to experience preterm birth (Chapter 3: Risk factors for spontaneous preterm birth); how women may be monitored more closely (Chapter 4: Specialist care for the woman at risk); the interventions she may be offered to prevent preterm birth (Chapter 5: Interventions to prevent spontaneous preterm birth) and reduce the

DOI: 10.4324/9781003380504-1

chance of her baby having problems if preterm birth cannot be prevented (Chapter 6: Interventions to improve neonatal outcomes). The handbook also covers the care of symptomatic women (Chapter 7: Care of the woman in threatened preterm labour), women admitted as inpatients (Chapter 8: Care of the woman in hospital) and a look to the future (Chapter 9: What the future may hold for preterm birth care). Although there is some reference to care of the newborn preterm baby, the focus is on the woman and neonatal care of her baby is beyond the scope of this book. It is written in an easy and accessible format, to support busy midwives in providing appropriate midwifery care. Although this book relates to maternity care in the UK, other midwives around the world may also find it useful.

What is preterm birth?

Defining preterm birth is not always as straightforward as one might think. Losing a wanted baby at any stage of pregnancy is profoundly distressing, and how this loss is referred to is very important, particularly to women and their families. If it happens before 14 weeks of pregnancy, the loss is described as an early or first trimester miscarriage, and between 14 and 23 weeks it is called a late miscarriage, or mid-trimester loss. In the UK, legal 'viability', when there is legal obligation to register the birth of a baby, whether live or stillborn, is 24 completed weeks of pregnancy. If a baby is born alive before 24 weeks, it is legally 'registrable' and may be described as a periviable preterm birth (see Figure 1.1).

The gestations at which babies are potentially viable are getting earlier and earlier. In 1990, the Abortion Act 1967 was amended to reduce legal viability from 28 to 24 weeks, but since then, babies have continued to survive at earlier gestations. The British Association of Perinatal Medicine's 'Perinatal Management of Extreme Preterm Birth before

	First trimester	Second trimester		Third trimester	
			Periviable		
Gestation in weeks	14	20	preterm birth 24	37	40
			(if live birth)		
Definition when pregnancy ends at this gestation	Early miscarriage or first trimester loss	Late miscarriage or mid-trimester loss (if the baby is stillborn)		Preterm birth (live birth or stillbirth)	Term birth

Figure 1.1 Pregnancy gestations and end of pregnancy definitions

27 weeks of gestation: A Framework for Practice' (British Association of Perinatal Medicine, 2019) demonstrates the chances of survival and severe disability for extremely preterm babies born alive (Figure 1.2) and recommends that active management may be considered from

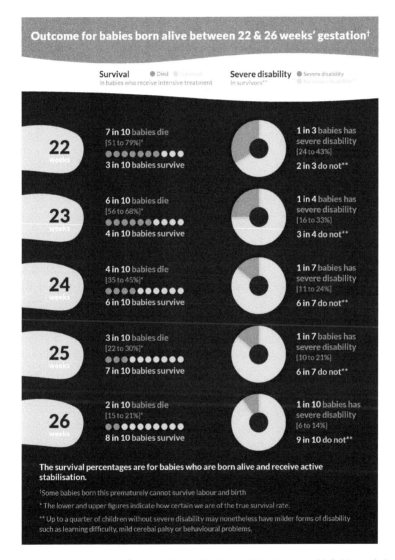

Figure 1.2 Infographic: 'Outcome for babies born alive between 22 & 26 weeks' gestation'

Source: From BAPM (2019), *reproduced with permission*

22^{+0} weeks, following assessment of risk and multiprofessional discussion with parents.

Definitions differ, not just over time, such as in the UK before and after 1990, but between countries. For example, in Australia a birth at 20 weeks' gestation is defined as a stillbirth, rather than a miscarriage (Australian Institute of Health and Welfare, 2023). This makes comparisons across time and countries, and epidemiological studies, difficult.

Why is addressing preterm birth important?

Preterm birth affects families worldwide. Globally, an estimated 0.94 million babies died from preterm birth complications in 2019 (Perin et al., 2022). The babies that do survive prematurity frequently have short- and long-term sequelae, such as cerebral palsy and developmental problems (Patel, 2016). In 2021, 7.6% of babies (approximately 47,000) in England and Wales were born preterm (Office for National Statistics, 2023). These are similar rates to Scotland where 6.5% of singleton babies were born preterm in 2021/22 (Public Health Scotland, 2022), and Northern Ireland where 7.8% of babies were born preterm in 2018/19 (Public Health Intelligence Unit, 2023). Preterm birth is estimated as costing health services £3.4 bn a year in England and Wales, and delaying preterm birth across all gestational groups by one week would save public services £994 million a year (Mangham *et al.*, 2009).

UK government targets and national policies

In November 2015, the UK Secretary of State for Health announced a target to reduce the rate of stillbirths, neonatal and maternal deaths by 50% by 2030 (Department of Health and Social Care, 2015). In order to help meet these targets for stillbirth and early neonatal death, the first version of *'Saving Babies Lives Care Bundle'*

(NHS England, 2016) was published. This care bundle included four elements (reducing smoking in pregnancy; risk assessment and surveillance for fetal growth restriction; raising awareness of reduced fetal movement; effective fetal monitoring during labour).

In 2017, the Department of Health published the 'Safer Maternity Care: progress and next steps' report (Department of Health, 2017). In this report, the national target of reducing the rate of stillbirths, neonatal and maternal deaths by 50%, was brought forward by five years to 2025. As premature birth is recognised as a major cause of neonatal mortality and morbidity (Perin *et al.*, 2022), the report also included the aim of reducing the preterm birth rate from 8% (of babies born preterm per year in England) to 6% by 2025. Following this, the *Saving Babies Lives Care Bundle* was revised to include a new fifth element on reducing preterm birth (NHS England, 2019). This was the first time national guidance formally mentioned providing care for asymptomatic women at high risk of preterm birth and specialist preterm birth surveillance clinics. The *Saving Babies Lives Care Bundle* has been further updated in 2023. This third version is discussed in more detail in Chapters 4 and 6, but a brief outline of the pathway is shown in Figure 1.3.

Saving Babies Lives Care Bundle (SBLCB) is an NHS England document, so the devolved nations of the UK are not obliged to implement it. However, elements of SBLCB that overlap with the NICE Preterm Birth Guidance (National Institute for Health and Care Excellence, 2015) will have influenced practice in Wales, Scotland and Northern Ireland.

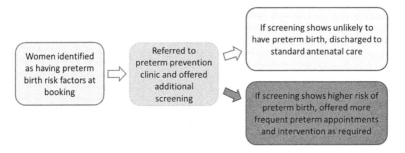

Figure 1.3 Outline of the preterm birth surveillance pathway recommended in *Saving Babies Lives Care Bundle* v.3

The role of the midwife in the care of women at risk of preterm birth

The role of the midwife in preterm birth care is developing rapidly, and the notion of a specialist midwifery role in preterm birth is still relatively new. In versions 2 and 3 of *Saving Babies Lives Care Bundle* (NHS England, 2019, 2023), the role of the midwife in providing preterm birth care is seen as pivotal. The pathway begins with midwives assessing the woman's risk of preterm birth at their first booking appointment. Appropriate antenatal care therefore hinges on their accurate assessment. The care bundle recommends that hospitals have a dedicated preterm birth team that includes a midwife lead (NHS England, 2023). The end of the pathway involves preparation for an anticipated preterm delivery, and midwives need to know about appropriate medications and interventions to ensure optimal outcomes for both mother and baby.

Midwives frequently care for women at risk of preterm at various stages of their pregnancy journey, and yet there is currently little focus on this issue during undergraduate midwifery training, and little specific post-registration training. This is the first book written by midwives for midwives on preterm birth, and we hope that you find it helpful in developing your understanding and confidence when caring for women at risk.

Use of preterm birth and mid-trimester loss terminology in this book

Whatever the definition, when a baby is born spontaneously at any gestation before 37 weeks, the physiological mechanisms involved are often similar (Ugwumadu, 2010). It follows, then, that the specialist care intended to prevent preterm birth can also prevent mid-trimester loss. The emotional consequences are also the same, and midwives should be mindful of this, particularly when talking to women about their current or previous experience of mid-trimester loss or preterm birth (see Box 1.1).

Box 1.1 In her own words: woman's experience of care during mid-trimester pregnancy loss

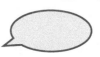

I am sure I was born broody because for as long as I can remember I longed to have a big family. Aged 25 and newly married, it seemed this dream was to become a reality.

Words cannot describe how much my first loss at 19 weeks' gestation crushed me; after all, I was supposed to be out of the woods by the second trimester. Besides, everyone knew I was pregnant, I had bought new baby clothes and was obsessed with tracking my pregnancy progress. The D&C process, I heard also being referred to as a 'womb scrape', felt brutal to my ears and only deepened my trauma. I learned how much language really matters in these moments – the word imagery was harrowing. After a long period of physical, mental and emotional recovery, somehow I was ready to try again.

Losing baby number 2 utterly devastated me. As well as being an anxious wreck throughout the second pregnancy, I also denied the tell-tale signs of spotting for as long as I could, putting off calling the local midwife team, instead I hoped and prayed against another loss. Sadly, after feeling a strong sensation to push, I went into labour on the toilet. I was 21 weeks pregnant. I remember the concerned looks on the paramedics' faces as they rushed me to the hospital where I had to complete the birthing process. The baby was stillborn but fully intact in his amniotic sac, greatly arousing the interest of the medical staff.

I accepted the free burial service offered to me which also significantly eased my grief. I was grateful to be able to say a proper goodbye to Joshua; it was much more dignifying as well. I recognised the importance of being treated with dignity in such undignifying circumstances, even small gestures made a difference, such as using the term 'baby' – it helped acknowledge the humanity of the child I almost had, and whose kicks were already causing my womb to flutter. I could not relate well to the term 'miscarriage', even 'late miscarriage' felt wrong, this was a fully-formed baby. I had lost my child.

I actually felt huge relief when a diagnosis was given for my condition. I still recall the lovely conversation with the obstetrician and how he sketched a little diagram clearly explaining the importance of cervical lengths during pregnancy. My weak cervix meant I should be a candidate for a cervical stitch and be treated as 'high risk' for future pregnancies.

Nzinga

It is important to note here that different terminology is sometimes used (for example mid-trimester loss, late miscarriage or second trimester miscarriage), and contentious terminology (for example incompetent cervix) throughout the literature. During the development of this book, we have taken advice from women with lived experience, and we have used the terminology they prefer.

Summary

In this first chapter, we have aimed to provide a background to spontaneous preterm birth, how common it is, its potential consequences and how the role of the midwife fits with current maternity care policy around care of women at risk.

Box 1.2 **Chapter summary and recommendations for practice**

- Nearly 8% of babies a year are born preterm in England and Wales, costing health services £3.4 bn annually.
- The frequency of preterm birth, combined with governmental drives (such as publication of NHS England's *Saving Babies Lives Care Bundle*, Element 5), means that all midwives now require a comprehensive understanding of preterm birth.
- Preterm birth and mid-trimester loss share similar aetiologies, so care is similar for both.
- This book aims to help midwives to increase their knowledge and confidence in caring for women at risk.

References

Australian Institute of Health and Welfare (2023) National Perinatal Mortality Data Collection, 2021; Quality Statement. Available online: https://meteor.aihw.gov.au/content/783855 Accessed: 20/04/2024.

British Association of Perinatal Medicine (2019) Perinatal Management of Extreme Preterm Birth Before 27 weeks of Gestation. A BAPM Framework for Practice. https://www.bapm.org/resources/80-perinatal-management-of-extreme-preterm-birth-before-27-weeks-of-gestation-2019 Accessed: 20/04/2024.

Carlisle, N., Dalkin, S., Shennan, A., & Sandall, J. 2024. IMplementation of the preterm birth surveillance PAthway: A RealisT evaluation (The IMPART study). *Implementation Science Communications*, 5(1), 57.

Department of Health and Social Care. (2015, November 13). *New ambition to halve rate of stillbirths and infant deaths.* https://www.gov.uk/government/news/new-ambition-to-halve-rate-of-stillbirths-and-infant-deaths Accessed: 24/04/2024.

Department of Health. (2017). *Safer Maternity Care - The National Maternity Safety Strategy - Progress and Next Steps.* Available online: https://www.gov.uk/government/publications/safer-maternity-care-progress-and-next-steps Accessed: 20/04/2024.

Goldenberg, R. L., Culhane, J. F., Iams, J. D., & Romero, R. 2008. Epidemiology and causes of preterm birth. *The Lancet*, 371(9606), 75–84. https://doi.org/10.1159/000314018

Mangham, L. J., Petrou, S., Doyle, L. W., Draper, E. S., & Marlow, N. (2009). The cost of preterm birth throughout childhood in England and Wales. *PEDIATRICS*. https://doi.org/10.1542/peds.2008-1827

NHS England. (2016). *Saving Babies' Lives A care bundle for reducing stillbirth.* Available online: https://www.england.nhs.uk/wp-content/uploads/2016/03/saving-babies-lives-car-bundl.pdf Accessed: 24/04/2024

NHS England. (2019). *Saving Babies Lives Care Bundle Version 2.* Available online: https://www.england.nhs.uk/wp-content/uploads/2019/07/saving-babies-lives-care-bundle-version-two-v5.pdf Accessed: 24/04/2024

NHS England. (2023) *Saving Babies Lives Care Bundle Version 3.* Available online: https://www.england.nhs.uk/wp-content/uploads/2023/05/PRN00614-Saving-babies-lives-version-three-a-care-bundle-for-reducing-perinatal-mortality.pdf Accessed: 20/04/2024

National Institute for Health and Care Excellence (2015). Preterm Labour and Birth. NICE guideline. Last updated June 2022. Available online: https://www.nice.org.uk/guidance/ng25 Accessed: 20/04/2024

Office for National Statistics (2023). *Birth characteristics in England and Wales: 2021.* Available online: https://www.ons.gov.uk/peoplepopulationandcommunity/birthsdeathsandmarriages/livebirths/bulletins/birthcharacteristicsinenglandandwales/2021 Accessed: 20/04/2024

Patel, R. M. (2016). Short- and long-term outcomes for extremely preterm infants. *American Journal of Perinatology*, 33(3), 318–328. https://doi.org/10.1055/s-0035-1571202

Perin, J., Mulick, A., Yeung, D., Villavicencio, F., Lopez, G., Strong, K. L., Prieto-Merino, D., Cousens, S., Black, R. E., & Liu, L. (2022 Feb 1). Global, regional, and national causes of under-5 mortality in 2000–19: An updated systematic analysis with implications for the sustainable development goals. *The Lancet*

Child & Adolescent Health, 6(2), 106–15. doi:10.1016/S2352-4642(21) 00311-4.

Public Health Intelligence Unit. (2023). *Children's Health in Northern Ireland: a statistical profile of births using data drawn from the Northern Ireland Child Health System, Northern Ireland Maternity System and Northern Ireland Statistics and Research Agency 2019/20.* Available online: https://www. publichealth.hscni.net/statistical-profile-childrens-health-northern-ireland-201920 Accessed: 20/04/2024

Public Health Scotland (2022). *Births in Scotland Year ending 31 March 2022*: A National Statistics release for Scotland. Available online: https:// publichealthscotland.scot/publications/births-in-scotland/births-in-scotland-year-ending-31-march-2022/ Accessed: 20/04/2024.

Ugwumadu, A. (2010). Chorioamnionitis and mid-trimester pregnancy loss. *Gynecologic and Obstetric Investigation*, 70(4), 281–285. https://doi.org/ 10.1159/000314018

Chapter 2
Causes of spontaneous preterm birth

Introduction

When a baby is born early, the first thing the woman wants to know is: why did it happen? Unfortunately, this question is not always easy to answer; we do not completely understand what causes labour at term, and the same is true at earlier gestations. Determining what caused this particular woman's labour is challenging, at least in part, because it is likely to have been multiple factors (Olson et al., 1995). Evidence suggests that labour is likely due to an inflammatory response triggered by a combination of factors (Areia and Mota-Pinto, 2022). These triggers include infection, hormone balances, uterine haemorrhage, uterine overdistension (stretch) and cervical insufficiency (Goldenberg et al., 2008; Romero et al., 2014). It could also be triggered by stress, by way of activation of the maternal/fetal hypothalamic-pituitary-adrenal axis (Duthie and Reynolds, 2013) or other signals from the fetus, such as cell-free DNA (Dugoff et al., 2016). These potential triggers are discussed in more detail below.

The second question women usually ask is whether anything could have been done to prevent it. The answer to this question is: possibly, yes, had we been able to predict it. Specialist preterm care focuses on assessing individual risk and offering interventions, when needed, to prevent preterm birth. Predictive tools and interventions used in preterm clinics are discussed in Chapter 4: Specialist care for the woman at risk and Chapter 5: Interventions to prevent spontaneous preterm birth.

DOI: 10.4324/9781003380504-2

Whether a cause can be identified or not, women need to be reassured that it is very unlikely that anything they did, or didn't do, caused them to deliver early. Having said that, individuals do have some control over modifiable factors and lifestyle choices that can affect their risk of preterm birth, such as smoking and using recreational drugs, so these need to be addressed, sensitively, as well.

Inflammation

What is inflammation, or the inflammatory response? Put simply, it is the response of the body's immune system which is designed to protect us from things that could be harmful, such as external pathogens and damaged cells that can lead to cancer. The immune system is made up of many different organs, cells and proteins, which include chemical messengers called cytokines. Cytokines activate other cells to do certain things, for example, they instruct large white blood cells to travel to areas of damage, whilst also increasing fluid between cells (oedema) which facilitates this movement, allowing elimination of pathogens.

In the case of labour, it is believed that pro-inflammatory cytokines, including, but by no means exclusively, interleukin 6 (IL-6) and interleukin 8 (IL-8), are responsible for activating a chain of events that lead to changes in the texture of the cervix (ripening) and cause uterine cells to contract/retract (Pandey et al., 2017; Park et al., 2005). This appears to be the case in both term and preterm labour. When considering the causes of preterm labour, the clinician needs to explore factors that may have triggered that immune response. Potential factors are discussed below.

Infection

The most obvious (and common) trigger that activates the inflammatory response in any human body is infection, and infection is associated with around 40% of preterm births (Boyle *et al.*, 2017).

The most common infections associated with preterm birth are genital tract infections, but others, intrauterine and systemic infections, can also trigger the inflammatory response that leads to preterm birth. Women who have Group B Streptococcus (GBS) and Trichomonas are more likely to experience preterm birth (Seale *et al.*, 2017; Van Gerwen *et al.*, 2021) as are those who have asymptomatic bacteriuria or recurrent urine infections (Werter *et al.*, 2021). When a woman has her baby early, often no pathogen is identified, and if one is identified, it may be subclinical, that is, one that has not caused any obvious signs or symptoms. However, any untreated systemic infection (Grette *et al.*, 2020) (Wang *et al.*, 2023; Yao *et al.*, 2022) poses an increased risk likely due to inflammatory cytokines which might trigger preterm labour pathways.

Bacterial vaginosis (BV) is not an infection in itself but occurs when the balance of natural bacteria in the vagina is disrupted, with potentially harmful bacteria predominating. It is associated with an increased risk of preterm birth (Mohanty *et al.*, 2023). It should be treated when it is found, however, universal screening of all pregnant women remains controversial (Bretelle *et al.*, 2023).

Although Candida (thrush) is common, sometimes recurring and can be difficult to eradicate in pregnancy, it is not associated with an increased risk of preterm birth (Schuster *et al.*, 2020).

The vaginal tract is not a sterile environment, but the presence of intact membranes usually keeps the fetus safe from ascending infection. Even if the membranes are intact, infection may make its way into the uterine cavity. The very length of the cervix, with its protective 'mucus plug' means ascending infection is less likely, but it is not always guaranteed. Once the inflammatory response has begun, it may or may not be dampened by the woman's physiology.

What we don't know is whether the pathogens causing the infection entered the uterine cavity first, and triggered the process, which led to cervical shortening, or whether the cervix shortened first, which made it easier for the pathogens to enter.

When a woman presents in preterm labour, and after a preterm birth, microbiology swabs are usually taken to investigate the presence of infection, and the placenta and membranes are often examined for signs of chorioamnionitis (inflammation of the fetal membranes). This doesn't tell us, however, whether the infection was the initial cause of the preterm labour or whether the ascending infection came after an initiation of labour and ruptured membranes. In many cases, though, and certainly in most term births, a pathogen cannot be identified. In preterm labour, there is no evidence for prescribing antibiotics blindly. Unless clinicians are treating something specific such as a urinary tract infection, it is important to remember that antibiotics may make the situation worse. For example, they may mask infection (Liu et al., 2001) or in the case of co-amoxiclav, can increase the risk of necrotising colitis in the neonate (Kenyon et al., 2002).

Over- or under-active immune response

Compromise of the woman's immune system could result in disruption of the delicate balance of protection from infection and over-activity of the immune response that triggers labour. Factors that could comprise the immune system include: lifestyle (e.g. smoking and poor nutrition), natural susceptibility to infection and stress (Barrea *et al.*, 2021; Jiang *et al.*, 2020; Maddock and Pariante, 2001). The stress associated with poverty and racism may account for the increased risk of poor pregnancy outcomes in women from socially deprived and ethnic minority groups (Shenassa *et al.*, 2021). Smoking and recreational drug use may also be more common in women living with stress, thereby compounding the problem.

The vaginal microbiome (the complex micro-ecosystem that makes up the vaginal flora) may also have a role to play in protecting women from infection. There is increasing evidence that women whose vaginal microbiome is dominated by colonies of the bacteria *Lactobacillus crispatus* are less likely to experience preterm birth (Bayar *et al.*, 2020).

Conversely, labour may be triggered by an over-active immune system. This could occur where there is a reduced materno-fetal tolerance. This is a modulation of the woman's immune system to protect the fetus (with half its genes being paternal) from rejection (Romero *et al.*, 2014). The mechanism is poorly understood, but there may be a genetic susceptibility to a reduced materno-fetal tolerance or the result of the relationship between both parents' genotypes.

Preterm birth is also more likely in women with auto-immune diseases, such as systemic lupus erythematosus (SLE) and anti-phospholipid syndrome (APS) (Kolstad *et al.*, 2020). Perhaps the body of a woman with APS has a lower threshold for the inflammatory response that triggers labour, as well as the thrombotic events associated with APS (Walter *et al.*, 2021).

Bleeding

Bleeding in early pregnancy is associated with mid-trimester loss and preterm birth (Yang *et al.*, 2004). Thrombin, an important clotting factor involved in the control of bleeding, can stimulate myometrial activity, and women with increased thrombin generation are at increased risk of spontaneous preterm birth (Romero *et al.*, 2014). This may explain the increased risk of preterm birth following trauma, either as a result of an accident, e.g. a road traffic accident, or deliberate injury, e.g. domestic violence, as well as in women with APS. This trauma could, of course, also be compounded by the stress associated with the event that caused it.

Cervical insufficiency

An important risk factor for preterm birth is cervical insufficiency (sometimes called 'cervical incompetence'). The role of the cervix in protecting from infection is discussed above, but preterm birth often follows a 'silent' shortening of the cervix, with no obvious signs or symptoms of labour until very late in the process, and where no pathogen is found. Certainly, chorioamnionitis is often found, but not in all cases. What triggers labour in these cases is harder to understand. Perhaps the inflammatory response is triggered by an unknown pathogen which our current tests cannot identify, as we know the risk of infection is higher when the cervix is short. Or perhaps the cervix has shortened and is opening because the inflammatory response has been triggered by something else? We do not know.

Cervical weakness may be naturally occurring, perhaps a family trait, which might at least partly explain the increased risk in women whose mothers or sisters experienced preterm birth (Koire *et al.*, 2021).

However, it may also be the result of cervical surgery, dilation and curettage (D&C) or previous in-labour caesarean section. These can undermine the integrity of the cervix, as can some medical conditions, including Ehlers-Danlos syndrome. Factors relating to cervical weakness are discussed in more detail in Chapter 3: Risk factors for spontaneous preterm birth.

Decline in progesterone action

During pregnancy, the hormone progesterone is vital for the woman's body to maintain the pregnancy. It is thought that a change in the ratio of oestrogen and progesterone hormones towards the end of pregnancy has a role in the change from a quiescent (quiet) uterus to one stimulated into labour by that inflammatory response (Romero *et al.*, 2014). Progesterone antagonists, such as mifepristone, are used in medical terminations of pregnancy. While the role of progesterone in preterm labour is uncertain, progesterone supplementation is a treatment given to women at risk (see Chapter 5: Interventions to prevent spontaneous preterm birth). However, it is possible that it works (for some women) because of its anti-inflammatory qualities, rather than in the maintenance of hormonal balance.

Overdistension of the uterus

Overdistension of the uterus, or stretch, also appears to have a role in initiating labour. This is seen in women at term, as well as at earlier gestations in multiple pregnancies and women with polyhydramnios (Goldenberg *et al.*, 2008). It is thought that this overstretching can lead to an inflammatory response that triggers labour (Waldorf *et al.*, 2015). This may be because of damage caused by stretching that the body is trying to repair. This could also be why women with uterine anomalies and Asherman's syndrome are more likely to experience preterm birth. Again, these factors are discussed in more detail in Chapter 3: Risk factors for spontaneous preterm birth.

Stress

As previously noted, stress is associated with an increased risk of preterm birth. This compounds the problem for women at high risk of preterm birth as they often experience considerable stress and anxiety throughout subsequent pregnancies (see Chapter 4: Specialist care for the woman at risk). A large body of literature suggests an association between stress and preterm birth and plausible aetiologies (such as the interaction between stress hormones and the inflammatory response), have been suggested (Christian, 2012; Latendresse, 2009; Rich-Edwards and Grizzard, 2005; Ruiz *et al.*, 2003; Wadhwa *et al.*, 2001). The form of stress may also be important. Lobel *et al.* (2008), in their study of 279 pregnant women, found that pregnancy-specific stress (e.g. concerns about the baby's health), may be an even more important contributor to adverse birth outcomes than general stress.

Signals from the baby

Labour may also be triggered by signalling from the fetus through activation of the maternal/fetal hypothalamic-pituitary-adrenal axis (a stress response, involving cortisol) (Duthie and Reynolds, 2013). It may also be triggered by cell-free fetal DNA (Gomez-Lopez *et al.*, 2020). This may occur when the fetus is ready to be born (at term) or, when preterm, the fetus is in danger from maternal inflammatory cytokines, which may be harmful for the fetal brain (Boyle *et al.*, 2017) as well as from infection itself.

Summary

In this chapter, we have described the known, and potential, causes of spontaneous preterm birth. It is likely that the actual cause of an individual woman's preterm labour is a combination of several factors. This contributes to making preterm birth difficult to predict and may explain why particular interventions work for some and not others. Perhaps the reason that the currently available interventions work, when they do, is in their effect on the immune system; cerclage and pessary may work because the woman's immune system recognises a foreign body and sends extra forces to the cervix to protect it from infection, although not enough to cause an over-reaction and trigger labour. Similarly, progesterone may work because it gives an extra boost of anti-inflammatory factors that are perhaps needed in, for example, women with a lower 'tolerance' to the fetus or a compromised immune system that has resulted from stress.

Potential causes of preterm birth and their relationship with associated risk factors are shown in Figure 2.1.

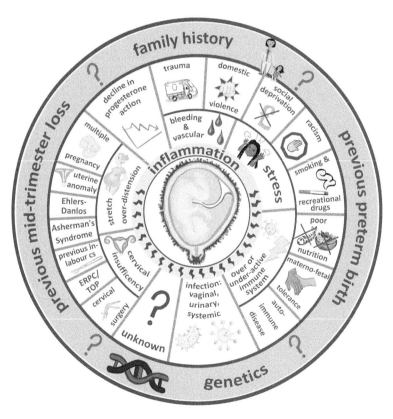

Figure 2.1 Potential causes of preterm birth and associations with risk factors

Artist: Gemma Baxter

Box 2.1 Chapter summary and recommendations
for practice

- Inflammation (inflammatory response) is a complicated mechanism that appears to start labour.
- This inflammatory response could be triggered by a number of factors or a combination of factors.
- Reasons for preterm birth should be investigated and explained to the parents as well as possible; women should be reassured they are unlikely to have done anything to have caused it.
- Determining what triggered previous preterm labour may help to guide future care to prevent it from happening again.
- Midwives should ensure women with previous preterm birth are referred to specialist preterm service in subsequent pregnancies.

References

Areia, A. L., & Mota-Pinto, A. 2022. Inflammation and preterm birth: A systematic review. *Reproductive Medicine*, *3*(2), 101–111. https://doi.org/10.1159/000314018

Barrea, L., Muscogiuri, G., Frias-Toral, E., Laudisio, D., Pugliese, G., Castellucci, B., Garcia-Velasquez, E., Savastano, S., & Colao, A. 2021. Nutrition and immune system: From the Mediterranean diet to dietary supplementary through the microbiota. *Critical Reviews in Food Science and Nutrition*, *61*(18), 3066–3090. https://doi.org/10.1159/000314018

Bayar, E., Bennett, P. R., Chan, D., Sykes, L., & MacIntyre, D. A. 2020, August. The Pregnancy Microbiome and Preterm Birth. In *Seminars in Immunopathology* (Vol. 42, pp. 487–499). Springer, Berlin Heidelberg.

Boyle, A. K., Rinaldi, S. F., Norman, J. E., & Stock, S. J. 2017. Preterm birth: Inflammation, fetal injury and treatment strategies. *Journal of Reproductive Immunology*, *119*, 62–66.

Bretelle, F., Loubière, S., Desbriere, R., Loundou, A., Blanc, J., Heckenroth, H., Schmitz, T., Benachi, A., Haddad, B., Mauviel, F., & Danoy, X. 2023. Effectiveness and costs of molecular screening and treatment for bacterial vaginosis to prevent preterm birth: The AuTop randomized clinical trial. *JAMA Pediatrics*, *177*(9), 894–902. https://doi.org/10.1159/000314018

Christian, L. M. 2012. Psychoneuroimmunology in pregnancy: Immune pathways linking stress with maternal health, adverse birth outcomes, and fetal development. *Neuroscience & Biobehavioral Reviews*, *36*(1), 350–361. https://doi.org/10.1159/000314018

Dugoff, L., Barberio, A., Whittaker, P. G., Schwartz, N., Sehdev, H., & Bastek, J. A. 2016. Cell-free DNA fetal fraction and preterm birth. *American Journal of Obstetrics and Gynecology*, *215*(2), 231–e1. https://doi.org/10.1159/000314018

Duthie, L., & Reynolds, R. M. 2013. Changes in the maternal hypothalamic-pituitary-adrenal axis in pregnancy and postpartum: Influences on maternal and fetal outcomes. *Neuroendocrinology*, *98*(2), 106–115. https://doi.org/10.1159/000314018

Goldenberg, R. L., Culhane, J. F., Iams, J. D., & Romero, R. 2008. Epidemiology and causes of preterm birth. *The Lancet*, *371*(9606), 75–84. https://doi.org/10.1159/000314018

Gomez-Lopez, N., Romero, R., Schwenkel, G., Garcia-Flores, V., Panaitescu, B., Varrey, A., Ayoub, F., Hassan, S. S., & Phillippe, M. 2020. Cell-free fetal DNA increases prior to labor at term and in a subset of preterm births. *Reproductive Sciences*, *27*, 218–232.

Grette, K., Cassity, S., Holliday, N., & Rimawi, B. H. 2020. Acute pyelonephritis during pregnancy: A systematic review of the aetiology, timing, and reported adverse perinatal risks during pregnancy. *Journal of Obstetrics and Gynaecology*, *40*(6), 739–748. https://doi.org/10.1159/000314018

Jiang, C., Chen, Q., & Xie, M., 2020. Smoking increases the risk of infectious diseases: A narrative review. *Tobacco Induced Diseases*, *18*.

Kenyon, S., Taylor, D. J., & Tarnow-Mordi, W. O.; ORACLE Collaborative Group. 2002. ORACLE—Antibiotics for preterm prelabour rupture of the membranes: Short-term and long-term outcomes. *Acta Paediatrica Supplement*, *91*(437):12–5. doi: 10.1111/j.1651-2227.2002.tb00153.x. PMID: 12200889.

Koire, A., Chu, D. M., & Aagaard, K. 2021. Family history is a predictor of current preterm birth. *American Journal of Obstetrics & Gynecology MFM*, *3*(1), 100277. https://doi.org/10.1159/000314018

Kolstad, K. D., Mayo, J. A., Chung, L., Chaichian, Y., Kelly, V. M., Druzin, M., Stevenson, D. K., Shaw, G. M., & Simard, J. F. 2020. Preterm birth phenotypes in women with autoimmune rheumatic diseases: A population-based cohort study. *BJOG: An International Journal of Obstetrics & Gynaecology*, *127*(1), 70–78. https://doi.org/10.1159/000314018

Latendresse, G. 2009. The interaction between chronic stress and pregnancy: Preterm birth from a biobehavioral perspective. *Journal of Midwifery and Women's Health*, *54*(1), 8–17. https://doi.org/10.1159/000314018

Liu, Y. C., Huang, W. K., Huang, T. S., & Kunin, C. M. 2001 Oct 22. Inappropriate use of antibiotics and the risk for delayed admission and masked diagnosis of infectious diseases: A lesson from Taiwan. *Archives of Internal Medicine*, *161*(19), 2366–2370. doi: 10.1001/archinte.161.19.2366. PMID: 11606153.

Lobel, M., Cannella, D. L., Graham, J. E., DeVincent, C., Schneider, J., & Meyer, B. A. 2008. Pregnancy-specific stress, prenatal health behaviors, and birth outcomes. *Health Psychology*, *27*(5), 604–615. https://doi.org/10.1159/000314018

Maddock, C., & Pariante, C. M. 2001. How does stress affect you? An overview of stress, immunity, depression and disease. *Epidemiology and Psychiatric Sciences*, *10*(3), 153–162. https://doi.org/10.1159/000314018

Mohanty, T., Doke, P. P., & Khuroo, S. R. 2023. Effect of bacterial vaginosis on preterm birth: A meta-analysis. *Archives of Gynecology and Obstetrics*, *308*(4), 1247–1255. https://doi.org/10.1159/000314018

Olson, D. M., Mijovic, J. E., & Sadowsky, D. W. 1995, February. Control of human parturition. *Seminars in Perinatology*, *19*(1), 52–63. WB Saunders. https://doi.org/10.1159/000314018

Pandey, M., Chauhan, M., & Awasthi, S. 2017 Sep. Interplay of cytokines in preterm birth. *Indian Journal of Medical Research*, *146*(3), 316–327. https://journals.lww.com/ijmr/fulltext/2017/46030/Interplay_of_cytokines_in_preterm_birth.5.aspx PMID: 29355137; PMCID: PMC5793465.

Park, J. S., Park, C. W., Lockwood, C. J., & Norwitz, E. R. 2005 August. Role of cytokines in preterm labor and birth. *Minerva Ginecol*, *57*(4), 349–66. PMID: 16170281.https://doi.org/10.1159/000314018

Rich-Edwards, J. W., & Grizzard, T. A. 2005. Psychosocial stress and neuroendocrine mechanisms in preterm delivery. *American Journal of Obstetrics and Gynecology*, *192*(5), S30–S35. https://doi.org/10.1159/000314018

Romero, R., Dey, S. K., & Fisher, S. J. 2014. Preterm labor: One syndrome, many causes. *Science*, *345*(6198), 760–765. https://doi.org/10.1159/000314018

Ruiz, R. J., Fullerton, J., & Dudley, D. J. 2003. The interrelationship of maternal stress, endocrine factors and inflammation on gestational length. *Obstetrical & Gynecological Survey*, *58*(6), 415–428. https://doi.org/10.1159/000314018

Schuster, H. J., de Jonghe, B. A., Limpens, J., Budding, A. E., & Painter, R. C. 2020. Asymptomatic vaginal Candida colonization and adverse pregnancy outcomes including preterm birth: A systematic review and meta-analysis. *American Journal of Obstetrics & Gynecology MFM*, *2*(3), 100163. https://doi.org/10.1159/000314018

Seale, A. C., Bianchi-Jassir, F., Russell, N. J., Kohli-Lynch, M., Tann, C. J., & Hall, J., *et al.* 2017. Estimates of the burden of group B streptococcal disease worldwide for pregnant women, stillbirths, and children. *Clinical Infectious Diseases*, *65*, S200–S219. doi: 10.1093/cid/cix664

Shenassa, E. D., Widemann, L. G., & Hunt, C. D. 2021. Antepartum depression and preterm birth: Pathophysiology, epidemiology, and disparities due to structural racism. *Current Psychiatry Reports*, *23*, 1–14.

Van Gerwen, O. T., Craig-Kuhn, M. C., Jones, A. T., Schroeder, J. A., Deaver, J., Buekens, P., Kissinger, P. J., & Muzny, C. A. 2021. Trichomoniasis and adverse birth outcomes: A systematic review and meta-analysis. *BJOG: An International Journal of Obstetrics & Gynaecology*, *128*(12), 1907–1915. https://doi.org/10.1159/000314018

Wadhwa, P. D., Culhane, J. F., Rauh, V., Barve, S. S., Hogan, V., Sandman, C. A., Hobel, C. J., Chicz-DeMet, A., Dunkel-Schetter, C., & Garite, T. J. 2001. Stress, infection and preterm birth: A biobehavioural perspective. *Paediatric and Perinatal Epidemiology*, *15*(s2), 17–29. https://doi.org/10.1159/000314018

Waldorf, K. M. A., Singh, N., Mohan, A. R., Young, R. C., Ngo, L., Das, A., Tsai, J., Bansal, A., Paolella, L., Herbert, B. R., & Sooranna, S. R. 2015. Uterine overdistention induces preterm labor mediated by inflammation: Observations in pregnant women and nonhuman primates. *American Journal of Obstetrics and Gynecology*, *213*(6), 830–e1. https://doi.org/10.1159/000314018

Walter, I. J., Haneveld, M. J. K., Lely, A. T., Bloemenkamp, K. W. M., Limper, M., & Kooiman, J. 2021. Pregnancy outcome predictors in antiphospholipid syndrome: A systematic review and meta-analysis. *Autoimmunity Reviews*, *20*(10), 102901. https://doi.org/10.1159/000314018

Wang, X., Ou, H., Wu, Y., & Xing, Z. 2023. Risk of preterm birth in maternal influenza or SARS-CoV-2 infection: A systematic review and meta-analysis. *Translational Pediatrics*, *12*(4), 631. https://doi.org/10.1159/000314018

Werter, D. E., Kazemier, B. M., Schneeberger, C., Mol, B. W., de Groot, C. J., Geerlings, S. E., & Pajkrt, E. 2021. Risk indicators for urinary tract infections in low risk pregnancy and the subsequent risk of preterm birth. *Antibiotics*, *10*(9), 1055. https://doi.org/10.1159/000314018

Yang, J., Hartmann, K. E., Savitz, D. A., Herring, A. H., Dole, N., Olshan, A. F., & Thorp, J. M. Jr. 2004. Vaginal bleeding during pregnancy and preterm birth. *American Journal of Epidemiology*, *160*(2), 118–125. https://doi.org/10.1159/000314018

Yao, X. D., Zhu, L. J., Yin, J., & Wen, J. 2022. Impacts of COVID-19 pandemic on preterm birth: A systematic review and meta-analysis. *Public Health*, *213*, 127–134.

Chapter 3

Risk factors for spontaneous preterm birth

Introduction

This chapter discusses the importance of preterm birth risk assessment for all women booking for maternity care and outlines the risk assessments and care pathways recommended in NHS England's *Saving Babies Lives Care Bundle* (SBLCBv3) (NHS England, 2023). The chapter goes on to explain many and varied risk factors for spontaneous preterm birth, which include previous preterm birth and mid-trimester pregnancy loss, cervical surgery, short cervical length, previous in-labour caesarean section, uterine abnormalities, multiple pregnancy, Asherman's and Ehlers-Danlos syndromes, as well as family history and demographic characteristics.

Preterm birth risk assessment

There are many reasons why a woman may be at risk of spontaneous preterm birth. In the absence of better methods of prediction, these 'risk factors' are used to determine who may benefit from additional care designed to reduce the chance of preterm birth. It is important to remember, however, that more than 50% of women who deliver preterm do not have any known risk factors (Iams *et al.*, 2001), and that approximately two-thirds of women with traditional risk factors do not deliver preterm (Nageotte *et al.*, 1994; Phillips *et al.*, 2017) (Figure 3.1).

DOI: 10.4324/9781003380504-3

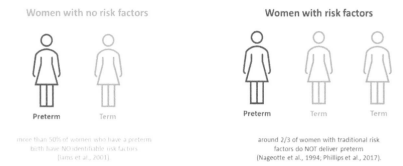

Figure 3.1 Prevalence of preterm birth in women with and without risk factors

As a minimum, NHS maternity services in England offer pregnant women a risk assessment and care pathway based on NHS England's SBLCBv3 Element 5, as summarised in Table 3.1.

NHS hospitals in devolved countries are not obliged to follow these guidelines but may choose to do so. Some hospitals in England may offer more than the minimum recommended. This often depends on local capacity. They may also be using an alternative method for risk assessment that has been agreed with their local commissioners and network. The risk factors listed in *Saving Babies Lives Care Bundle*, along with some additional factors, are explained in detail throughout this chapter.

Previous preterm birth or mid-trimester loss (late miscarriage)

A prior preterm delivery or mid-trimester pregnancy loss is the most predictive risk factor for subsequent preterm birth or mid-trimester loss in the next pregnancy (Edlow *et al.*, 2007; Ferrero *et al.*, 2016; Sneider *et al.*, 2016). If a woman has had a previous preterm birth, her risk of having another preterm birth is approximately four to six times greater than if she hasn't had a previous baby born early (Ferrero *et al.*, 2016). The risk increases with each early delivery, e.g. women with two previous preterm births are at greater risk than women with one previous preterm birth. The risk is also higher when the preterm birth or mid-trimester loss occurs at earlier gestational ages, e.g. a woman with a previous delivery at 24 weeks' gestation has a

Table 3.1 Summary of risk factors and care recommendations for asymptomatic women at risk of preterm birth

Level of risk	Risk factor	Care pathway	
		Surveillance	Management
High	• Previous preterm birth or mid-trimester loss (16–34 weeks' gestation). • Previous preterm prelabour rupture of membranes. • Previous use of cervical cerclage. • Known uterine variant (i.e. unicornuate, bicornuate uterus or uterine septum). • Intrauterine adhesions (Asherman's syndrome). • History of trachelectomy (for cervical cancer).	1. Referral to local or tertiary preterm prevention clinic by 12 weeks. 2. Further risk assessment based on history +/− examination as appropriate in secondary care with identification of pregnant women needing referral to tertiary services. 3. All pregnant women are to be offered transvaginal cervix scanning every 2–4 weeks between 16 and 24 weeks as a secondary test to more accurately quantify the risk of preterm birth. 4. Additional use of quantitative fetal fibronectin in asymptomatic pregnant women may be considered where centres have this expertise.	Interventions should be offered to pregnant women as appropriate, based on either history or additional risk assessment tests by clinicians able to discuss the relevant risks and benefits according to up-to-date evidence and relevant guidance, for example UK Preterm Clinical Network guidance and NICE guidance. These interventions should include cervical cerclage, pessary and progesterone as appropriate.

(Continued)

(Continued)

Level of risk	Risk factor	Care pathway	
		Surveillance	Management

Intermediate	• Previous birth by caesarean section at full dilatation.
	• History of significant cervical excisional event, i.e. LLETZ where >15 mm depth removed, or >1 LLETZ procedure carried out or cone biopsy (knife or laser, typically carried out under general anaesthetic).
		1. Refer to preterm birth prevention clinic by 12 weeks.
		2. Further risk assessment based on history +/- examination as appropriate in secondary care with discussion of option of additional risk assessment tests, including:
		  a. A single transvaginal cervix scan between 18 and 22 weeks as a minimum.
		  a. Additional use of quantitative fetal fibronectin in asymptomatic pregnant women can be considered where centres have this expertise.
			1. Interventions should be discussed with pregnant women as appropriate based on either history or additional risk assessment tests by clinicians able to discuss the relevant risks and benefits according to up-to-date evidence and relevant guidance. These interventions should include cervical cerclage, pessary and progesterone as appropriate.
			2. Pregnant women at intermediate risk should be reassessed at 24 weeks for consideration of transfer back to a low-risk pathway.

Source: Adapted from SBLCBv3 Appendix F: Risk assessment, surveillance pathway and management of women at risk of preterm birth.

higher risk of recurrence than a woman with a previous delivery at 34 weeks (Iams and Berghella, 2010; McManemy *et al.*, 2007).

It can be challenging when women present with a mixed history of both term and preterm births. This is because women with a prior term pregnancy are frequently considered to have a decreased risk of subsequent spontaneous preterm birth. One study found that the outcome of the third pregnancy is more likely to be correlated to the outcome of the second pregnancy, rather than the first (Ouh *et al.*, 2018). However, another paper found there was a higher risk of preterm birth in women who had both term and spontaneous preterm births, compared to women who had experienced only previous spontaneous preterm births (Suff, Xu, Dalla Valle, *et al.*, 2022). This seems counter-intuitive but may be explained by events that occurred in the term birth, for example, an in-labour caesarean section, which is discussed in more detail below.

The relationship between risk and previous experience of preterm birth is clearly important, which underlines the need for the booking midwife to take a careful history. This history should include not just gestations at birth of previous babies but the circumstances in which they occurred, and if any causes had been suggested, e.g. infection or in-labour caesarean section. This is discussed in more detail in Chapter 4: Specialist care for the woman at risk.

Cervical surgery

Invasive cervical surgery increases the risk of preterm birth, although midwives may have developed little awareness of this in their practice. This is understandable, as gynaecology is not a major element of midwifery training (Carlisle *et al.*, 2024). Yet understanding the different types of cervical surgery and how they affect risk of preterm birth is important because midwives need to know when to refer the women in their care for specialist review. In this section, we explain why cervical surgery is sometimes needed, the different types of surgery and their implications for future pregnancies.

Cervical screening

Cervical screening is known to substantially reduce deaths from cervical cancer (Wilailak *et al.*, 2021). This screening (sometimes called a 'smear test' or 'pap smear') began in the UK in 1964, aiming to identify changes in cervical cells that could lead to cancer. Treatments, if required, can then be offered earlier and are therefore more likely to be effective.

This screening aims to identify abnormal cells, which are described as cervical intraepithelial neoplasia (CIN). CIN is not cancer itself, but if left untreated, these cells could develop into cervical cancer over time. These changes are often only found when a woman undergoes cervical screening as CIN does not cause any symptoms (Macmillan Cancer Support, 2021). The main causes of CIN are the human papillomavirus (HPV) and smoking.

If abnormal cells are found, the woman will usually be invited for a colposcopy (using a microscope called a colposcope to look closely at the cervix). This may take place at her local hospital gynaecology or colposcopy clinic. A small biopsy (called a 'cervical punch biopsy') may also be undertaken at the same time. This is a very small amount of tissue, and this procedure does not increase a woman's risk of preterm birth.

Treatments for CIN and cervical cancer

CIN is graded into three categories, as shown in Table 3.2, along with treatment options (Macmillan Cancer Support, 2021).

Treatments for CIN 2 and CIN 3 vary internationally (Sasieni *et al.*, 2016). In some countries cone biopsy is recommended, in others laser therapy and/or large loop excision of the transformation zone (LLETZ) (Sasieni *et al.*, 2016). LLETZ is sometimes referred to as a loop

Table 3.2 Grades of cervical intraepithelial neoplasia (CIN), extent of cervical tissue involvement and treatment options

CIN grade	Area of cervix affected	Treatment options
CIN 1	One-third of the thickness of the cervical surface layer is affected by abnormal cells.	This often returns to normal without any treatment; however, the woman will probably be offered further cervical smear tests or colposcopies to ensure the cells have improved.
CIN 2	Two-thirds of the thickness of the cervical surface layer is affected by abnormal cells.	Often treatment, or another colposcopy, is offered.
CIN 3	The full thickness of the cervical surface layer is affected by abnormal cells.	Treatment will be offered.

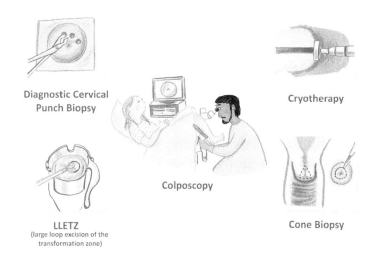

Diagnostic Cervical
Punch Biopsy

Cryotherapy

Colposcopy

LLETZ
(large loop excision of the
transformation zone)

Cone Biopsy

Figure 3.2 Some of the cervical investigations and treatments that may be carried out in a colposcopy clinic

Artist: Gemma Baxter

electrosurgical excision procedure (LEEP) or loop diathermy. Some common cervical procedures and treatments are shown in Figure 3.2.

If cervical cancer itself is detected, the options for treatment depend on the stage of the cancer. Early stage cervical cancers which are contained within the cervix (stage 1A–1B) can be treated through a LLETZ procedure, a cone biopsy or through more invasive surgery, such as a trachelectomy or hysterectomy (Table 3.3). Chemotherapy, radiotherapy and other treatments may be offered to women diagnosed with cervical cancer that has spread outside the cervix to nearby areas (stages 1B2–4A) and advanced cervical cancers which have spread outside the pelvis (stage 4B) (Jo's Trust, 2020). Treatments for cervical cancer can affect fertility which may be a concern for women who are planning future pregnancies. These women may be offered treatment that aims to preserve their fertility (sometimes called 'fertility preservation treatment'), or they may be referred to a fertility specialist to discuss other options such as egg or embryo freezing (Jo's Trust, 2020).

The more invasive the procedure, the greater the chance of preterm birth in subsequent pregnancies. Although the risk of preterm birth is increased by excisions of less than 10 mm in depth, this risk could be almost twofold for excisions of more than 10 mm, threefold for more

Table 3.3 Procedures for cervical screening and treatments with type of analgesia or anaesthetic usually offered

Procedure or treatment	Description	Analgesia or anaesthetic offered
Cervical screening test (smear or Pap test)	A speculum is inserted into the vaginal, and a special brush is rotated in the cervical canal to collect cells and test for HPV virus.	None.
Colposcopy	Using a microscope called a colposcope to look closely at the cervix.	None.
Diagnostic cervical punch biopsy	Small biopsy of cervix to determine if the woman needs further treatment.	None or local anaesthetic.
Cold coagulation	A probe is placed onto any areas with abnormal cells to burn them away.	None or local anaesthetic.
Cryotherapy	A probe is used to freeze the abnormal cells.	None or local anaesthetic.
'Large loop excision of the transformation zone' (LLETZ), also known as 'loop electrosurgical excision' (LEEP), or 'loop diathermy'	A thin wire loop is used to remove the transformation zone (which is the area around the opening of the cervix).	Local anaesthetic if smaller areas are removed. General anaesthetic or sedation if larger area of the cervix is removed.
'Needle excision of the transformation zone' (NETZ)	Similar to a LLETZ but the thin wire used is straight rather than a loop.	Sedation and/or local or general anaesthetic depending on area removed.
Laser therapy/laser ablation	A laser beam is used to burn away the abnormal cells.	Sedation and/or local or general anaesthetic depending on area being treated.
Cone biopsy/cold knife cone biopsy/ knife excision/ surgical knife	A minor operation where a cone-shaped wedge of tissue from the cervix is removed.	Usually under general anaesthetic.
Trachelectomy	Surgery to remove the cervix. Women planning future pregnancies may be offered transabdominal cerclage (TAC) (see Chapter 5).	General anaesthetic.
Hysterectomy	Surgery to remove the uterus (and cervix).	General anaesthetic.

than 15–17 mm and nearly fivefold for excisions exceeding 20 mm in depth (Kyrgiou et al., 2016). Deeper and larger excisions are usually undertaken under general anaesthetic.

Important questions to ask about a woman's experience of cervical screening and treatment are shown in Table 3.4.

Table 3.4 Questions to ask women about their experience of cervical screening and treatments, with suggested responses

Question	Suggested response
Have you ever had cervical screening (smear, Pap test)?	If 'No': tell her that cervical screening is very important and ask her to consider making an appointment with her GP or practice nurse after she has had the baby.
	If 'Yes': ask her what the result was and document what she says. If normal, reassure, if further investigations and/or treatments were carried out, ask the additional questions below.
	If 'Unsure': show her a speculum. This can help when explaining the procedure. She may not know what a 'smear test' is but is likely to remember having a speculum examination.
Have you had any procedures or treatment on your cervix?	If 'Yes': ask the below questions.
What cervical procedures or treatments did you have?	Document as described. If she does not know what it was called, ask her to explain what happened. Reference to Table 3.3 may be helpful.
What pain relief or anaesthetic, if any, did you have?	Document as described. This is especially useful in helping you to assess whether a 'biopsy' was a simple punch biopsy or a more invasive cone biopsy, which is often carried out under general anaesthetic.
Do you know how much cervix was removed?	Document as described. If she doesn't know, ask her where the procedure was carried out; you may be able to contact the hospital to find out. If you remain unsure, refer her to the preterm clinic.
When was the treatment carried out?	Document as described. Knowing whether it was before or after any previous pregnancies, and when those pregnancies ended will help the preterm clinic to determine her risk in this pregnancy.
What was the follow up/ was any further treatment needed?	Document as described.

Following these questions, if she is eligible, or you are unsure, refer her to your specialist preterm clinic.

Short cervical length

Cervical length, measured during a transvaginal ultrasound scan (TVUS), has been shown to identify women at higher risk of preterm birth, and the shorter the cervical length, the higher the risk (Berghella *et al.*, 1997; Crane and Hutchens, 2008; de Carvalho *et al.*, 2005; Honest *et al.*, 2003). Cervical length screening for all pregnant women is not currently recommended by NICE or NHS England. This is because cervical length screening is not sufficiently accurate in nulliparous women (Esplin et al., 2017). Although there is ongoing debate as to whether it should be offered to all, and particularly those having their first baby, there is global consensus that it should be offered to those with known risk factors (Dawes *et al.*, 2020; Medley *et al.*, 2018). The procedure is explained in detail in Chapter 4: Specialist care for the woman at risk.

Measurement of cervical length is standard practice in specialist preterm clinics, so this is where the majority of short cervixes are identified. However, they are occasionally detected as incidental findings during other ultrasound scans, e.g. during the 20-week anomaly scan. In these cases, women are often referred to a specialist preterm clinic for confirmation and further investigation.

The thresholds at which a cervix is considered 'short' varies between different clinicians, hospitals and countries. In the UK, the most commonly used threshold, at between 14 and 24 weeks' gestation, is 25 mm, i.e. a cervix is considered short at 24 mm or less (Dawes *et al.*, 2020). This is because this threshold relates to the 10th percentile in this gestational category (Owen *et al.*, 2001). However, current NICE guidance recommends using a cervical length of 25 mm or less (National Institute for Health and Care Excellence, 2015). In addition to cervical length, other features that are associated with increased risk of preterm birth may be noted on ultrasound (such as the presence of a funnel and amniotic fluid 'sludge'). These are discussed in more detail in Chapter 4: Specialist care for the woman at risk.

Once a hospital has appropriately trained staff and equipment, TVUSs are comparatively cheap to perform. However, there is currently a shortage of clinicians trained in this skill. This may be, at least in part, because transvaginal ultrasound assessment of cervical length is not yet included in the core Royal College of Obstetrics and Gynaecologists (RCOG) curriculum (RCOG, 2022). It is a skill that can be learned by midwives, but similarly it is not a core competency (Sholapurkar *et al.*, 2021).

Previous caesarean section in labour

Evidence has shown an association between mid-trimester loss and spontaneous preterm birth in women with a previous in-labour caesarean section (Cong *et al.*, 2018; Levine *et al.*, 2015; Wang *et al.*, 2020). The closer to full dilatation at caesarean, the greater the risk of subsequent preterm birth (Williams *et al.*, 2021). Women with a previous caesarean at 9 or 10 cm were 2.48 times more likely to have a subsequent spontaneous preterm birth, compared to 1.63 times more likely if the caesarean had been undertaken at 0–4 cm dilated (Barros *et al.*, 2018; Wood *et al.*, 2017). Although this association with preterm birth has only relatively recently been identified, previous caesarean section at full dilatation is now recognised as risk factor for preterm birth in *Saving Babies Lives Care Bundle* (NHS England, 2023) and women with this history should be referred for review by a specialist preterm clinic.

The physiological mechanism behind this increased risk is currently believed to be cervical damage caused by an unintentionally low uterine incision (Mckelvey *et al.*, 2010). This arises because as the cervix effaces during labour, it becomes continuous with the lower segment of the uterus, and therefore a lower segment caesarean section (LSCS) incision may damage cervical tissue within (Figure 3.3). This explains why the risk is highest at full dilatation. The more dilated the cervix, the more cervical tissue will have been drawn up into the lower segment of the uterus. Additionally, women undergoing caesarean sections at full dilatation are more likely to experience intra-operative trauma, e.g. lacerations to the uterine artery, bladder, bowel or ureter, and extension of the uterine incision (Allen *et al.*, 2005). This disruption and scarring of cervical tissue are thought to result in cervical weakness in future pregnancies, hence the increased risk of future mid-trimester loss and spontaneous preterm birth.

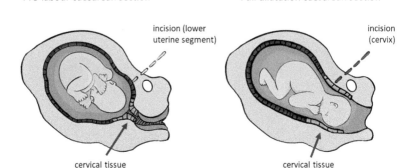

Pre-labour caesarean section   Full dilatation caesarean section

incision (lower uterine segment)   incision (cervix)

cervical tissue   cervical tissue

Figure 3.3 Caesarean section incision sites before labour and at full dilatation

Source: Images reproduced with kind permission of Andrew Shennan, artist: Georgie Proctor

There is an even higher risk of recurring spontaneous preterm birth in women who have had a spontaneous preterm birth after an emergency caesarean section. Research has shown that in women who have had an emergency caesarean section at term (at any stage of labour) and have a subsequent spontaneous preterm birth, 54% go on to have another preterm birth. This is compared to 20% of women with a prior spontaneous preterm birth but not an emergency caesarean section (Suff, Xu, Glazewska-Hallin, *et al.*, 2022). It also appears that vaginally placed cerclage, a treatment for preventing preterm birth, is less effective in these women (Hickland *et al.*, 2020). This is discussed in more detail in Chapter 5: Interventions to prevent spontaneous preterm birth. Research further exploring in-labour caesarean as a risk factor for preterm birth is underway (Carlisle *et al.*, 2020).

Uterine abnormalities

Women who were born with uterine anomalies are more likely to experience preterm birth. These anomalies are sometimes referred to as congenital Müllerian anomalies, after Johannes Müller, a physiologist who first described the Müllerian duct in 1830. The duct, which is seen in both female and male embryos, develops into the female reproductive tract when sexual differentiation occurs in the fetus. Müllerian anomalies include a spectrum of abnormalities which occur during Müllerian duct development. The degree of increased risk of miscarriage and preterm birth depends on the variant of the anomaly (Chan *et al.*, 2011; Mastrolia *et al.*, 2018; Reichman *et al.*, 2009). The most common variants are described and illustrated in Figure 3.4.

Illustration	Müllerian variant	Description
	Bicornuate uterus	A bicornuate uterus has an indentation at the top, meaning it is heart-shaped in appearance. Women with a bicornuate uterus have a slightly higher risk of miscarriage and preterm birth.
	Arcuate Uterus	An arcuate uterus has a slight dip at the fundus. It is thought that an arcuate uterus does not increase risk of preterm birth or early miscarriage, but it may increase risk of late miscarriage.
	Septate Uterus	A septate uterus is one uterus that is divided by a band of tissue. In some, this tissue runs the full length of the uterus, but in others, it only affects a section of the uterus. There is an increased risk of miscarriage and preterm birth.
	Unicornuate Uterus	A unicornuate uterus is when only half of the uterus has formed, resulting in a small, banana-shaped uterus. There is an increased risk of ectopic pregnancy, late miscarriage and preterm birth.
	Uterus Didelphys	Uterus didelphys, which is sometimes referred to as a double uterus, has various forms, e.g. some women have two uteruses, two cervixes and one vaginal, while others have two uteruses, cervixes, and two vaginas. These women have a small increase in the risk of preterm birth.

Figure 3.4 Congenital Müllerian anomalies of the female reproductive tract

Asherman's and Ehlers-Danlos syndromes

Asherman's syndrome and Ehlers-Danlos syndrome are known to increase the risk of spontaneous preterm birth. In Asherman's syndrome scar tissue, also described as intrauterine adhesions, builds up inside the uterus and/or cervix. It is a rare condition and most often develops after uterine surgery, such as dilation and curettage (D&C) procedures, or infection (usually severe pelvic infections, and less commonly tuberculosis and schistosomiasis). Studies have reported a preterm birth rate amongst women with Asherman's syndrome of between 17.9% and 50% (Baradwan *et al.*, 2018; McComb and Wagner, 1997; Yu *et al.*, 2008; Zikopoulos, 2004).

Ehlers-Danlos syndromes are a group of inherited conditions that affect connective tissues. In pregnancy and childbirth, the body and its tissues have to adapt considerably to the growth and birth of a baby (Pezaro *et al.*, 2021), so in some cases the disruption to normal physiology seen in Ehlers-Danlos syndromes can result in spontaneous preterm birth (Anum *et al.*, 2009; Karthikeyan and Venkat-Raman, 2018; Spiegel *et al.*, 2022).

Multiple pregnancy

The aetiology of spontaneous preterm births in multiple pregnancies is likely to be multifactorial, distinct from singleton pregnancies, and largely remains unidentified (Murray *et al.*, 2018). Different suggested mechanisms include intrauterine infection, cervical insufficiency and amplified uterine stretch/distension (Murray *et al.*, 2018).

Approximately 60% of twins are born preterm, with around a third due to spontaneous preterm labour and around 10% due to preterm rupture of membranes (Ananth and Chauhan, 2012). The remainder are iatrogenic preterm deliveries. Approximately 94.5% of triplets are born preterm (Kalikkot Thekkeveedu *et al.*, 2021).

Family history

Spontaneous preterm birth is associated with a maternal family history of preterm birth, i.e. female relatives within three generations. If a nulliparous woman was herself born preterm (i.e. her mother experienced preterm birth), she is 1.75 times more likely to deliver her baby preterm. If a woman's sister has had a preterm birth, she is 2.25 times more likely to have a preterm baby herself (Koire *et al.*, 2021). That said, this risk factor alone is not usually a specific criterion for referral to specialist preterm birth services. This is largely because preterm services have limited capacity and must focus their attention on those most at risk.

Demographic characteristics

Women with certain demographic characteristics are more likely to experience preterm birth. These include ethnicity (women from ethnic minority groups) and those living in deprived areas (Burgos Ochoa *et al.*, 2021; DeHority *et al.*, 2020; Kalikkot Thekkeveedu *et al.*, 2021; Li *et al.*, 2019; Mehra *et al.*, 2019; Puthussery *et al.*, 2019).

There is no evidence to suggest that the physiology of women from ethnic minority groups or socially deprived groups results in early birth, so these demographic 'risk factors' for preterm birth are markers for something else such as stress, poverty, racism, anxiety or pollution. There is nothing intrinsic about being black African which makes a woman more likely to have a preterm baby than a white British woman. In fact, studies have shown that women from minoritised ethnic backgrounds have similar or lower rates of preterm birth if they were foreign-born, compared to if they were born in the US or UK (Datta-Nemdharry *et al.*, 2012; Elo *et al.*, 2014; Li *et al.*, 2019; Puthussery *et al.*, 2019).

Lifestyle and other factors

Other lifestyle and social factors, such as smoking, use of recreational drugs and being at risk of domestic violence, are associated with increased risk of preterm birth but are not so significant as to warrant referral to specialist preterm clinics as per *Saving Babies Lives Care Bundle* criteria. They do, however, require referral to other specialist services, and midwives should be mindful that the woman who is already at high risk could be more so in these circumstances. D&C procedures and termination of pregnancy (TOP) also increase risk of preterm birth (Lemmers *et al.*, 2016). This is thought to be due to damage to the cervix, but again, women with this risk factor alone are not usually referred for specialist preterm surveillance.

Summary

In this chapter we have aimed to provide a comprehensive explanation of the most important risk factors for spontaneous preterm birth. We have not attempted to cover every possible factor that has been associated with increased risk. If you 'google' 'what is a risk factor for preterm birth?', you will be presented with a plethora of associated factors, but more research needs to be done to ascertain precisely how much they affect risk, both on their own and in combination with others.

Box 3.1 **Chapter summary and recommendations for practice**

- More than 50% of women who deliver preterm do not have any risk factors.
- Approximately two-thirds of women with traditional risk factors do not go on to deliver preterm.
- Midwives must ensure they take a detailed history at the booking appointment, to aid future care planning and referral to specialist preterm birth services when necessary.

References

Allen, V. M., O'Connell, C. M., & Baskett, T. F. (2005). Maternal and perinatal morbidity of caesarean delivery at full cervical dilatation compared with caesarean delivery in the first stage of labour. *BJOG: An International Journal of Obstetrics & Gynaecology*, *112*(7), 986–990. https://doi.org/10.1111/j.1471-0528.2005.00615.x

Ananth, C. V., & Chauhan, S. P. (2012). Epidemiology of twinning in developed countries. *Seminars in Perinatology*, *36*(3), 156–161. https://doi.org/10.1053/j. semperi.2012.02.001

Anum, E. A., Hill, L. D., Pandya, A., & Strauss, J. F. (2009). Connective tissue and related disorders and preterm birth: Clues to genes contributing to prematurity. *Placenta*, *30*(3), 207–215. https://doi.org/10.1016/j.placenta. 2008.12.007

Baradwan, S., Baradwan, A., Bashir, M., & Al-Jaroudi, D. (2018). The birth weight in pregnant women with Asherman syndrome compared to normal intrauterine cavity. *Medicine*, *97*(32), e11797.

Barros, F. C., Rabello Neto, D. de L., Villar, J., Kennedy, S. H., Silveira, M. F., Diaz-Rossello, J. L., & Victora, C. G. (2018). Caesarean sections and the prevalence of preterm and early-term births in Brazil: Secondary analyses of national birth registration. *BMJ Open*, *8*(8), e021538. https://doi.org/10.1136/ bmjopen-2018-021538

Berghella, V., Tolosa, J. E., Kuhlman, K., Weiner, S., Bolognese, R. J., & Wapner, R. J. (1997). Cervical ultrasonography compared with manual examination as a predictor of preterm delivery. *American Journal of Obstetrics & Gynecology*, *177*(4), 723–730. https://doi.org/10.1016/S0002-9378(97)70259-X

Burgos Ochoa, L., Bertens, L. C. M., Garcia-Gomez, P., van Ourti, T., Steegers, E. A. P., & Been, J. V. (2021). Association of neighbourhood socioeconomic trajectories with preterm birth and small-for-gestational-age in the Netherlands: A nationwide population-based study. *The Lancet Regional Health – Europe*, *10*. https://doi.org/10.1016/j.lanepe.2021.100205

Carlisle, N., Glazewska-Hallin, A., Story, L., Carter, J., Seed, P. T., Suff, N., Giblin, L., Huller, J., Napolitano, R., Rutherford, M., Alexander, D. C., Simpson, N., Banerjee, A., David, A. L., & Shennan, A. H. (2020). CRAFT (Cerclage after full dilatation caesarean section): Protocol of a mixed methods study investigating the role of previous in-labour caesarean section in preterm birth risk. *BMC Pregnancy and Childbirth*, *20*(1), 698. https://doi.org/10.1186/ s12884-020-03375-z

Carlisle, N., Dalkin, S., Shennan, A., & Sandall, J. (2024). IMplementation of the preterm birth surveillance PAthway: A RealisT evaluation (The IMPART study). *Implementation Science Communications*, *5*(1), 57.

Chan, Y. Y., Jayaprakasan, K., Tan, A., Thornton, J. G., Coomarasamy, A., & Raine-Fenning, N. J. (2011). Reproductive outcomes in women with congenital uterine anomalies: A systematic review. *Ultrasound in Obstetrics & Gynecology*, *38*(4), 371–382. https://doi.org/10.1002/uog.10056

Cong, A., de Vries, B., & Ludlow, J. (2018). Does previous caesarean section at full dilatation increase the likelihood of subsequent spontaneous preterm birth? *Australian and New Zealand Journal of Obstetrics and Gynaecology*, *58*(3), 267–273. https://doi.org/10.1111/ajo.12713

Crane, J. M. G., & Hutchens, D. (2008). Use of transvaginal ultrasonography to predict preterm birth in women with a history of preterm birth. *Ultrasound in Obstetrics & Gynecology*, *32*(5), 640–645. https://doi.org/10.1002/uog.6143

Datta-Nemdharry, P., Dattani, N., & Macfarlane, A. J. (2012). Birth outcomes for African and Caribbean babies in England and Wales: Retrospective analysis of routinely collected data. *BMJ Open*, *2*(3), e001088. https://doi.org/10.1136/bmjopen-2012-001088

Dawes, L., Groom, K., Jordan, V., & Waugh, J. (2020). The use of specialised preterm birth clinics for women at high risk of spontaneous preterm birth: A systematic review. *BMC Pregnancy and Childbirth*, *20*(1), 58. https://doi.org/10.1186/s12884-020-2731-7

de Carvalho, M. H. B., Bittar, R. E., Brizot, M. de L., Bicudo, C., & Zugaib, M. (2005). Prediction of preterm delivery in the second trimester. *Obstetrics & Gynecology*, *105*(3). https://journals.lww.com/greenjournal/Fulltext/2005/03000/Prediction_of_Preterm_Delivery_in_the_Second.15.aspx

DeHority, R. L., Coyne, K. D., Bevan, G. H., & Lappen, J. R. (2020). The relationship between social deprivation and preterm birth [OP03-7C]. *Obstetrics & Gynecology*, *135*. https://journals.lww.com/greenjournal/Fulltext/2020/05001/The_Relationship_Between_Social_Deprivation_and.18.aspx

Edlow, A. G., Srinivas, S. K., & Elovitz, M. A. (2007). Second-trimester loss and subsequent pregnancy outcomes: What is the real risk? *American Journal of Obstetrics and Gynecology*, *197*(6), 581.e1–581.e6. https://doi.org/10.1016/j.ajog.2007.09.016

Elo, I. T., Vang, Z., & Culhane, J. F. (2014). Variation in birth outcomes by mother's country of birth among non-Hispanic black women in the United States. *Maternal and Child Health Journal*, *18*(10), 2371–2381. https://doi.org/10.1007/s10995-014-1477-0

Esplin, M. S., Elovitz, M. A., Iams, J. D., Parker, C. B., Wapner, R. J., Grobman, W. A., Simhan, H. N., Wing, D. A., Haas, D. M., Silver, R. M., Hoffman, M. K., Peaceman, A. M., Caritis, S. N., Parry, S., Wadhwa, P., Foroud, T., Mercer, B. M., Hunter, S. M., Saade, G. R., … Network, for the nuMoM2b. (2017). Predictive accuracy of serial transvaginal cervical lengths and quantitative vaginal fetal fibronectin levels for spontaneous preterm birth among nulliparous women. *JAMA*, *317*(10), 1047–1056. https://doi.org/10.1001/jama.2017.1373

Ferrero, D. M., Larson, J., Jacobsson, B., di Renzo, G. C., Norman, J. E., Martin, J. N., Jr., D'Alton, M., Castelazo, E., Howson, C. P., Sengpiel, V., Bottai, M., Mayo, J. A., Shaw, G. M., Verdenik, I., Tul, N., Velebil, P., Cairns-Smith, S.,

Rushwan, H., Arulkumaran, S., ... Simpson, J. L. (2016). Cross-country individual participant analysis of 4.1 million singleton births in 5 countries with very high human development index confirms known associations but provides no biologic explanation for 2/3 of all preterm births. *PLOS ONE, 11*(9), e0162506-. https://doi.org/10.1371/journal.pone.0162506

Hickland, M. M., Story, L., Glazewska-Hallin, A., Suff, N., Cauldwell, M., Watson, H. A., Carter, J., Duhig, K. E., & Shennan, A. H. (2020). Efficacy of transvaginal cervical cerclage in women at risk of preterm birth following previous emergency cesarean section. *Acta Obstetricia et Gynecologica Scandinavica, 99*(11), 1486–1491. https://doi.org/10.1159/000314018

Honest, H., Bachmann, L. M., Coomarasamy, A., Gupta, J. K., Kleijnen, J., & Khan, K. S. (2003). Accuracy of cervical transvaginal sonography in predicting preterm birth: A systematic review. *Ultrasound in Obstetrics & Gynecology, 22*(3), 305–322. https://doi.org/10.1002/uog.202

Iams, J. D., & Berghella, V. (2010). Care for women with prior preterm birth. *American Journal of Obstetrics and Gynecology, 203*(2), 89–100. https://doi.org/10.1016/j.ajog.2010.02.004

Iams, J. D., Goldenberg, R. L., Mercer, B. M., Moawad, A. H., Meis, P. J., Das, A. F., Caritis, S. N., Miodovnik, M., Menard, M. K., Thurnau, G. R., Dombrowski, M. P., & Roberts, J. H. (2001). The preterm prediction study: Can low-risk women destined for spontaneous preterm birth be identified? *American Journal of Obstetrics & Gynecology, 184*(4), 652–655. https://doi.org/10.1067/mob.2001.111248

Jo's Trust. (2020). *Treatment Options for Cervical Cancer.* https://www.jostrust.org.uk/information/cervical-cancer/treatments/options

Kalikkot Thekkeveedu, R., Dankhara, N., Desai, J., Klar, A. L., & Patel, J. (2021). Outcomes of multiple gestation births compared to singleton: Analysis of multicenter KID database. *Maternal Health, Neonatology and Perinatology, 7*(1), 15. https://doi.org/10.1186/s40748-021-00135-5

Karthikeyan, A., & Venkat-Raman, N. (2018). Hypermobile Ehlers–Danlos syndrome and pregnancy. *Obstetric Medicine, 11*(3), 104–109. https://doi.org/10.1177/1753495X18754577

Koire, A., Chu, D. M., & Aagaard, K. (2021). Family history is a predictor of current preterm birth. *American Journal of Obstetrics & Gynecology MFM, 3*(1). https://doi.org/10.1016/j.ajogmf.2020.100277

Kyrgiou, M., Athanasiou, A., Paraskevaidi, M., Mitra, A., Kalliala, I., Martin-Hirsch, P., Arbyn, M., Bennett, P., & Paraskevaidis, E. (2016). Adverse obstetric outcomes after local treatment for cervical preinvasive and early invasive disease according to cone depth: Systematic review and meta-analysis. *BMJ, 354*, i3633. https://doi.org/10.1136/bmj.i3633

Lemmers, M., Verschoor, M. A. C., Hooker, A. B., Opmeer, B. C., Limpens, J., Huirne, J. A. F., Ankum, W. M., & Mol, B. W. M. (2016). Dilatation and curettage increases the risk of subsequent preterm birth: A systematic review and meta-analysis. *Human Reproduction*, *31*(1), 34–45. https://doi.org/10.1093/humrep/dev274

Levine, L. D., Sammel, M. D., Hirshberg, A., Elovitz, M. A., & Srinivas, S. K. (2015). Does stage of labor at time of cesarean delivery affect risk of subsequent preterm birth? *American Journal of Obstetrics and Gynecology*, *212*(3), 360.e1–360.e7. https://doi.org/10.1016/j.ajog.2014.09.035

Li, Y., Quigley, M. A., Macfarlane, A., Jayaweera, H., Kurinczuk, J. J., & Hollowell, J. (2019). Ethnic differences in singleton preterm birth in England and Wales, 2006-12: Analysis of national routinely collected data. *Paediatric and Perinatal Epidemiology*, *33*(6), 449–458. https://doi.org/10.1111/ppe.12585

Macmillan Cancer Support. (2021). *Cervical Intra-Epithelial Neoplasia (CIN)*. https://www.macmillan.org.uk/cancer-information-and-support/worried-about-cancer/pre-cancerous-and-genetic-conditions/cin

Mastrolia, S. A., Baumfeld, Y., Hershkovitz, R., Yohay, D., Trojano, G., & Weintraub, A. Y. (2018). Independent association between uterine malformations and cervical insufficiency: A retrospective population-based cohort study. *Archives of Gynecology and Obstetrics*, *297*(4), 919–926. https://doi.org/10.1007/s00404-018-4663-2

McComb, P., & Wagner, B. L. (1997). Simplified therapy for Asherman's syndrome. *Fertility and Sterility*, *68*(6), 1047–1050. https://doi.org/10.1159/000314018

Mckelvey, A., Ashe, R., Mckenna, D., & Roberts, R. (2010). Caesarean section in the second stage of labour: A retrospective review of obstetric setting and morbidity. *Journal of Obstetrics and Gynaecology*, *30*(3), 264–267. https://doi.org/10.3109/01443610903572109

McManemy, J., Cooke, E., Amon, E., & Leet, T. (2007). Recurrence risk for preterm delivery. *American Journal of Obstetrics and Gynecology*, *196*(6), 576.e1–576.e7. https://doi.org/10.1016/j.ajog.2007.01.039

Medley, N., Poljak, B., Mammarella, S., & Alfirevic, Z. (2018). Clinical guidelines for prevention and management of preterm birth: A systematic review. *BJOG: An International Journal of Obstetrics & Gynaecology*, *125*(11), 1361–1369. https://doi.org/10.1111/1471-0528.15173

Mehra, R., Shebl, F. M., Cunningham, S. D., Magriples, U., Barrette, E., Herrera, C., Kozhimannil, K. B., & Ickovics, J. R. (2019). Area-level deprivation and preterm birth: Results from a national, commercially-insured population. *BMC Public Health*, *19*(1), 236. https://doi.org/10.1186/s12889-019-6533-7

Murray, S. R., Stock, S. J., Cowan, S., Cooper, E. S., & Norman, J. E. (2018). Spontaneous preterm birth prevention in multiple pregnancy. *The Obstetrician & Gynaecologist*, *20*(1), 57–63. https://doi.org/10.1111/tog.12460

Nageotte, M. P., Casal, D., & Senyei, A. E. (1994). Fetal fibronectin in patients at increased risk for premature birth. *American Journal of Obstetrics & Gynecology*, *170*(1), 20–25. https://doi.org/10.1016/S0002-9378(94)70376-0

National Institute for Health and Care Excellence. (2015). *Preterm Labour and Birth. NICE Guideline*. Last updated June 2022. Available online: https://www.nice.org.uk/guidance/ng25. Accessed: 20/04/2024.

NHS England. (2023) *Saving Babies Lives Care Bundle Version 3*. Available online: https://www.england.nhs.uk/wp-content/uploads/2023/05/PRN00614-Saving-babies-lives-version-three-a-care-bundle-for-reducing-perinatal-mortality.pdf. Accessed: 20/04/2024.

Ouh, Y.-T., Park, J. H., Ahn, K. H., Hong, S.-C., Oh, M.-J., Kim, H.-J., Han, S. W., & Cho, G. J. (2018). Recurrent risk of preterm birth in the third pregnancy in Korea. *Journal of Korean Medical Science*, *33*(24). https://doi.org/10.3346/jkms.2018.33.e170

Owen, J., Yost, N., Berghella, V., Thom, E., Swain, M., Dildy, G. A., III, Miodovnik, M., Langer, O., Sibai, B., & McNellis, D. (2001). Mid-trimester endovaginal sonography in women at high risk for spontaneous preterm birth. *JAMA*, *286*(11), 1340–1348. https://doi.org/10.1001/jama.286.11.1340

Pezaro, S., Pearce, G., & Reinhold, E. (2021). A clinical update on hypermobile Ehlers-Danlos syndrome during pregnancy, birth and beyond. *British Journal of Midwifery*, *29*(9). https://www.britishjournalofmidwifery.com/content/clinical-practice/a-clinical-update-on-hypermobile-ehlers-danlos-syndrome-during-pregnancy-birth-and-beyond/

Phillips, C., Velji, Z., Hanly, C., & Metcalfe, A. (2017). Risk of recurrent spontaneous preterm birth: A systematic review and meta-analysis. *BMJ Open*, *7*(6), e015402. https://doi.org/10.1136/bmjopen-2016-015402

Puthussery, S., Li, L., Tseng, P.-C., Kilby, L., Kapadia, J., Puthusserry, T., & Thind, A. (2019). Ethnic variations in risk of preterm birth in an ethnically dense socially disadvantaged area in the UK: A retrospective cross-sectional study. *BMJ Open*, *9*(3), e023570. https://doi.org/10.1136/bmjopen-2018-023570

RCOG. (2022). *Ultrasound Training: Introduction*. RCOG Website. https://www.rcog.org.uk/careers-and-training/training/curriculum/subspecialty-training-curriculum/ultrasound-module-intermediate-ultrasound-of-early-pregnancy-complications/ultrasound-training-introduction/delivery-of-ultrasound-training/

Reichman, D., Laufer, M. R., & Robinson, B. K. (2009). Pregnancy outcomes in unicornuate uteri: A review. *Fertility and Sterility*, *91*(5), 1886–1894. https://doi.org/10.1016/j.fertnstert.2008.02.163

Sasieni, P., Castanon, A., Landy, R., Kyrgiou, M., Kitchener, H., Quigley, M., Poon, L. C. Y., Shennan, A., Hollingworth, A., Soutter, W. P., Freeman-Wang, T., Peebles, D., Prendiville, W., & Patnick, J. (2016). Risk of preterm birth following surgical treatment for cervical disease: Executive summary of a recent symposium. *BJOG: An International Journal of Obstetrics & Gynaecology, 123*(9), 1426–1429. https://doi.org/10.1111/1471-0528.13839

Sholapurkar, S., O'Brien, S., & Ficquet, J. (2021). Use of ultrasound in the antenatal space. *British Journal of Midwifery, 29*(7), 370–374.

Sneider, K., Christiansen, O. B., Sundtoft, I. B., & Langhoff-Roos, J. (2016). Recurrence of second trimester miscarriage and extreme preterm delivery at 16–27 weeks of gestation with a focus on cervical insufficiency and prophylactic cerclage. *Acta Obstetricia et Gynecologica Scandinavica, 95*(12), 1383–1390. https://doi.org/10.1111/aogs.13027

Spiegel, E., Nicholls-Dempsey, L., Czuzoj-Shulman, N., & Abenhaim, H. A. (2022). Pregnancy outcomes in women with Ehlers-Danlos syndrome. *The Journal of Maternal-Fetal & Neonatal Medicine, 35*(9), 1683–1689. https://doi.org/10.1080/14767058.2020.1767574

Suff, N., Xu, V. X., Dalla Valle, G., Carter, J., Brennecke, S., & Shennan, A. (2022). Prior term delivery increases risk of subsequent recurrent preterm birth: An unexpected finding. *Australian and New Zealand Journal of Obstetrics and Gynaecology, 62*(4), 500–505. https://doi.org/10.1111/ajo.13504

Suff, N., Xu, V. X., Glazewska-Hallin, A., Carter, J., Brennecke, S., & Shennan, A. (2022). Previous term emergency caesarean section is a risk factor for recurrent spontaneous preterm birth; a retrospective cohort study. *European Journal of Obstetrics and Gynecology and Reproductive Biology, 271*, 108–111. https://doi.org/10.1016/j.ejogrb.2022.02.008

Wang, M., Kirby, A., Gibbs, E., Gidaszewski, B., Khajehei, M., & Chua, S. C. (2020). Risk of preterm birth in the subsequent pregnancy following caesarean section at full cervical dilatation compared with mid-cavity instrumental delivery. *Australian and New Zealand Journal of Obstetrics and Gynaecology, 60*(3), 382–388. https://doi.org/10.1111/ajo.13058

Wilailak, S., Kengsakul, M., & Kehoe, S. (2021). Worldwide initiatives to eliminate cervical cancer. *International Journal of Gynecology & Obstetrics, 155*, 102–106.

Williams, C., Fong, R., Murray, S. M., & Stock, S. J. (2021). Caesarean birth and risk of subsequent preterm birth: A retrospective cohort study. *BJOG: An International Journal of Obstetrics & Gynaecology, 128*(6), 1020–1028. https://doi.org/10.1111/1471-0528.16566

Wood, S. L., Tang, S., & Crawford, S. (2017). Cesarean delivery in the second stage of labor and the risk of subsequent premature birth. *American Journal of Obstetrics and Gynecology, 217*(1), 63.e1–63.e10. https://doi.org/10.1016/j.ajog.2017.03.006

Yu, D., Li, T.-C., Xia, E., Huang, X., Liu, Y., & Peng, X. (2008). Factors affecting reproductive outcome of hysteroscopic adhesiolysis for Asherman's syndrome. *Fertility and Sterility, 89*(3), 715–722. https://doi.org/10.1016/j.fertnstert.2007.03.070

Zikopoulos, K. 2004. Live delivery rates in subfertile women with Asherman's syndrome after hysteroscopic adhesiolysis using the resectoscope or the Versapoint system. *Reproductive BioMedicine Online, 8*(6), 720–725. https://doi.org/10.1159/000314018

Chapter 4
Specialist care for the woman at risk

Introduction

In this chapter, specialist preterm care of the woman at high risk of preterm birth is described. This includes the questions she may be asked as part of her initial assessment and the monitoring procedures she may be offered. This may consist of: transvaginal ultrasound scans for cervical length measurement, fetal fibronectin testing and other predictive and biomarker tests and infection screening. This chapter provides the information midwives need to confidently support women who have been referred for specialist care, as well as guidance for midwives involved in setting up and managing a specialist preterm surveillance clinic in their own maternity service. The interventions women may be offered to reduce their risk of preterm birth are discussed in detail in Chapter 5: Interventions to prevent spontaneous preterm birth.

Initial assessment

A good initial assessment (history taking) is fundamental to providing individualised care (Boyd and Heritage, 2006). In the specialist preterm surveillance clinic, the history taking should be comprehensive and holistic, but will naturally focus on factors that influence the woman's risk of preterm birth. These factors are described in the following subsections.

DOI: 10.4324/9781003380504-4

Obstetric history

The most significant risk factor for preterm birth, as explained in Chapter 3: Risk factors for spontaneous preterm birth, is a history of preterm birth or mid-trimester loss, and many women referred for specialist preterm care will have experienced this. It is important to ask the gestation at which each pregnancy ended, and the circumstances around it, as these will provide clues to the possible cause and inform the planning of care for this pregnancy. This conversation should be undertaken with sensitivity, as recalling these details may be upsetting. The woman should be asked about all pregnancies, but more information is required about any spontaneous mid-trimester losses or preterm births. If the baby was named, make a note of this and refer to them by this name when exploring the circumstances around their birth. Questions to ask include: How did the miscarriage or labour start? Was it with pain, bleeding or rupture of membranes? Or did the baby come quickly with little warning? This could help the clinician to evaluate whether the birth was a result of cervical insufficiency. Was there any sign of infection, in her or the baby, placenta or membranes (chorioamnionitis)? Were there any other investigations, and what was she told may have been the cause, if any was suspected? How were her previous babies born: spontaneously, by forceps or ventouse or caesarean section (CS)? If she had a CS, was it before labour (elective) or in labour (not just whether it was an emergency CS, as these can occur before labour)? If in labour, at what stage, or dilatation? Did she have any specialist preterm surveillance in any previous pregnancies, and if so, was observation all that was required, or did she also have any interventions, such as cerclage or progesterone supplementation?

In terms of her current pregnancy, it is important to note whether this is a singleton or multiple pregnancy. Twins and higher multiples are much more likely to be born earlier than singletons, but if the woman has additional risk factors these babies may be born even earlier than they would otherwise have been.

Medical history

An understanding of the woman's wider medical history will also help to determine her risk of preterm birth, including medical conditions and prior surgery. Of particular importance is to determine whether she has had invasive cervical surgery, for example, following cervical screening. She may also report uterine anomalies, or Asherman's or Ehlers-Danlos syndromes. Please refer to Chapter 3: Risk factors for spontaneous preterm birth for detailed information on the most common risk factors for spontaneous preterm birth.

Mental wellbeing

Many women, especially those with experience of preterm birth or mid-trimester loss, are very anxious and may be struggling to cope with their feelings. Their mental wellbeing should be assessed at the initial and subsequent appointments, and referrals should be made, if necessary, for additional support, e.g. perinatal mental health specialists, NHS Talking Therapies (formerly known as IAPT) or their GP. Services vary around the country, but midwives should know what services are available locally and know how to refer women to them. It may be useful to implement a formal method of mental wellbeing screening, perhaps with widely used and validated tools, such as the GAD7 and PHQ9 questions, shown in Figure 4.1 (Kroenke *et al.*, 2001; Spitzer *et al.*, 2006). Women attending for specialist preterm surveillance clinic appointments can be asked to complete these questions on arrival, so they can be reviewed before the consultation. These questionnaires can be completed electronically, for example, some trusts enable women to complete them via their mobile phones after scanning a QR code, which then uploads their answers to their hospital records. This will allow the clinician to be prepared to have a conversation about how the woman is coping and to offer any additional support, if required.

Addressing mental wellbeing is important not just from a general wellbeing perspective, but because anxiety is associated with an increased risk of preterm birth. Improving mental health may, therefore, also reduce the woman's chance of having her baby early. A large body of evidence suggests an association between stress and increased risk of preterm birth (see Chapter 2: Causes of spontaneous preterm birth).

Other factors

Other factors, such as family history of preterm birth or mid-trimester loss, lifestyle factors, as well as recreational drug use and experience of domestic violence are also important. These should be ascertained with care and

PHQ9 (Patient Health Questionnaire) Assessment

Over the last 2 weeks, how often have you been bothered by any of the following problems?

		Not at all	Several days	More than half the days	Nearly every day
1	Little interest or pleasure in doing things	0	1	2	3
2	Feeling down, depressed, or hopeless	0	1	2	3
3	Trouble falling or staying asleep, or sleeping too much	0	1	2	3
4	Feeling tired or having little energy	0	1	2	3
5	Poor appetite or overeating	0	1	2	3
6	Feeling bad about yourself — or that you are a failure or have let yourself or your family down	0	1	2	3
7	Trouble concentrating on things, such as reading the newspaper or watching television	0	1	2	3
8	Moving or speaking so slowly that other people could have noticed? Or the opposite — being so fidgety or restless that you have been moving around a lot more than usual	0	1	2	3
9	Thoughts that you would be better off dead or of hurting yourself in some way	0	1	2	3

If you have had any of these problems, how difficult have they made it for you to do your work, take care of things at home, or get along with other people?

Not difficult at all   Somewhat difficult   Very difficult   Extremely difficult

GAD7 (Generalised Anxiety Disorder Assessment)

Over the last 2 weeks, how often have you been bothered by any of the following problems?

		Not at all	Several days	More than half the days	Nearly every day
1	Feeling nervous, anxious or on edge	0	1	2	3
2	Not being able to stop or control worrying	0	1	2	3
3	Worrying too much about different things	0	1	2	3
4	Trouble relaxing	0	1	2	3
5	Being so restless that it is hard to sit still	0	1	2	3
6	Becoming easily annoyed or irritable	0	1	2	3
7	Feeling afraid as if something awful might happen	0	1	2	3

Figure 4.1 Mental wellbeing assessment questions from the PHQ9 (Patient Health Questionnaire) (Kroenke *et al.*, 2001) and GAD7 (Generalised Anxiety Disorder) Assessments (Spitzer *et al.*, 2006)

sensitivity, just as they should during any other maternity appointment. For more details, see Chapter 3: Risk factors for spontaneous preterm birth.

After taking the woman's history, the clinician should explain the procedures and interventions, if any, that she will be offered, and she should be given the opportunity to ask questions. These procedures are explained in detail below. It is important for all midwives to have an

---

Box 4.1 In her own words: woman's experience of specialist preterm care

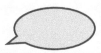

'I can't tell you how grateful we are to the team at the preterm clinic. If it weren't for them, we would never have gone on to have our two beautiful boys.

We were frightened to try again after losing our first two babies to preterm labour. For our last pregnancy (our daughter) our local midwife hadn't referred us to a specialist preterm clinic – something I really wish I had known to ask for, or that the midwife had known to refer us.

After we lost our daughter, we managed to get a referral to a London hospital via my GP. After some tests, we were told we had the all-clear to try again. However, I found the consultant who dealt with us at this hospital very cold and uncaring, and we just didn't have the confidence to try again based on what she had told us. Honestly, if this had been the only place we'd gone to we wouldn't have tried again. The way doctors and midwives speak to their patients just makes the biggest difference. She was so dismissive, she read our notes and just said "I'm not impressed with your situation." Maybe she meant to be reassuring, but it didn't come across that way!!

I heard about a specialist preterm clinic, at a different London hospital, by chance – on a Radio 4 programme, and I contacted them direct as a last hope. We were lucky enough to be invited for an appointment. To have a world-leading doctor in their field sit and just listen to us, what we'd been though and give their professional advice on what we should do, and then to invite us to come to their clinic for a cervical suture so the team could look after us, just meant so much to us. They were very kind and approachable. This made all the difference to us.

When I did become pregnant, we came back to the clinic and they arranged the cervical suture. I was very scared because of the risk of miscarriage. The team were lovely and reassuring. What really made a big difference was that they asked my opinion about the procedure; up until then, at the other hospitals, we had not been part of the decision-making process, and everything that had been done to us was someone else's decision. So that meant such a lot to us.

We came back for checkups every month or two, for fetal fibronectin tests and scans, which was amazing, for our peace of mind. To know that the baby was developing, growing well, and that I wasn't about to go into preterm labour, really helped.'

Claire M

understanding of these procedures, as women in their care may have questions before or after their preterm surveillance clinic appointments.

Cervical length measurement

Transvaginal ultrasound assessment of cervical length is currently the most common test offered to asymptomatic high-risk women as part of their preterm monitoring (Carlisle *et al.*, 2023). There is a strong body of evidence suggesting that the shorter the cervix, the more likely the baby will be born early. You can read more about short cervical length in Chapter 3: Risk factors for spontaneous preterm birth. In the UK, a threshold of 25 mm is recommended by the National Institute for Health and Care Excellence (NICE) (2015). What happens before, during and after a transvaginal ultrasound scan for measuring cervical length is explained in the subsections below.

Preparation for the scan

Before the procedure, the woman should be asked to empty her bladder. This is because a full bladder can put pressure on the cervix and make it appear longer than it is, giving false reassurance. She will need to remove her lower garments and underwear, so attention must be given to the protection of her privacy and dignity. The woman should be reassured that the scan will not harm the baby or increase the risk of miscarriage and that she can tell the sonographer to stop at any time. Any vaginal swabs, whether for fetal fibronectin testing or other investigations, should be taken before scan. The attending clinician should always remember the possibility that the woman undergoing this procedure may have experienced undisclosed sexual abuse.

The cervical length scan procedure

The ultrasound scan procedure is carried out using a special vaginal probe over several minutes. The cervix is part of the uterus and, like muscle tissue, its overall length can fluctuate. The cervical canal is visualised on the ultrasound screen from the internal to external os, and at least three measurements are taken, in millimetres, with the shortest measurement used to guide practice. Most cervixes of normal length,

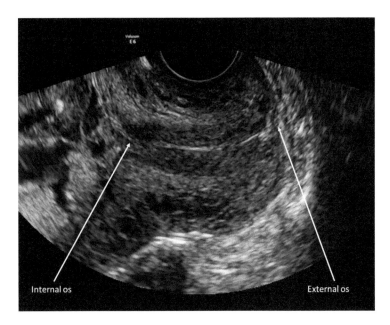

Internal os

External os

Figure 4.2 Transvaginal ultrasound scan image of a normal-length cervix

Source: Reproduced with kind permission of a preterm surveillance clinic patient

like the one shown in Figure 4.2, are curved, so the most accurate measurement will follow the curve. However, sometimes a straight line is drawn from internal to external os. This method may slightly underestimate the true length of the cervix, but this is preferred to over-estimating it. It is not usually an issue with short cervixes as they tend to be straight.

A transvaginal ultrasound scan image of a short cervix is shown in Figure 4.3. This image also shows 'funneling' which occurs when a weak internal os has started to open. The funnel's length and width are also usually measured, but it is the length of the closed cervix that is used for decision-making and predicting preterm birth with tools such as the QUiPP App.

Other factors that may be noted on the scan are: 'pressure effect' where fundal pressure is applied to mimic the additional pressure that could, for example, occur when the woman was standing; amniotic fluid 'sludge', which is thought to be a sign of inflammation, but its significance is not fully understood (Suff *et al.*, 2023); 'length above the stitch' is noted if there is a cerclage *in situ*; position and features of a previous CS scar, i.e. distance from the internal os, length, depth and width of a

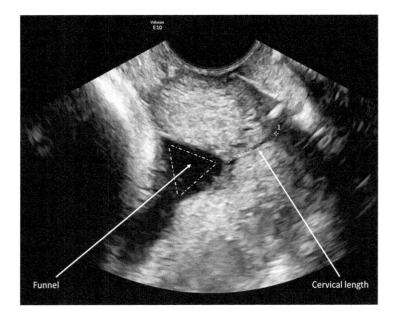

Figure 4.3 Transvaginal ultrasound scan image of a short cervix with funneling
Source: Reproduced with kind permission of a preterm surveillance clinic patient

scar niche, if this is seen. These CS scar characteristics appear to affect the likelihood of mid-trimester loss and preterm birth, but more research is needed to quantify this (Banerjee *et al.*, 2022).

After the cervical length scan

Although examination of the fetus is not the focus of the preterm clinic appointment, women are often offered the opportunity to 'see' their baby on a transabdominal scan. This can provide welcome additional reassurance. Some clinicians prefer to visualise the fetal heartbeat prior to commencing a cervical length scan, while others leave the choice to the woman.

Fetal fibronectin testing

Nearly half (49%) of hospitals responding to Carlisle and colleagues' (2023) survey offer fetal fibronectin (fFN) testing to asymptomatic high-risk women during specialist preterm surveillance. Fetal fibronectin is a natural protein found in amniotic fluid, placental tissue and in the decidua basilis of the placenta. It is believed to be released following mechanical or inflammatory damage to the membranes and its potential as a predictive marker for preterm birth, particularly its high negative predictive value (i.e. accuracy of a negative result), has been established for several years (Abbott *et al.*, 2013; Honest *et al.*, 2002; Leitich *et al.*, 1999; Lockwood *et al.*, 1991; Matsuura *et al.*, 1988; Peaceman *et al.*, 1997).

In the UK, test results for fFN were, until relatively recently, presented as dichotomous, (i.e. positive or negative), based on a threshold of 50 ng/ml. Newer analysers now provide results as concentrations of fetal fibronectin in ng/ml, and it has been suggested that using alternative thresholds or limits, i.e. <10 and >200 ng/ml, rather than a cut-off of 50 ng/ml, may improve positive prediction (i.e. accuracy of a positive result) of the test and further aid clinical management (Abbott *et al.*, 2013; Foster and Shennan, 2014).

Preparation for fetal fibronectin testing

An explanation of the procedure and how the result will help to guide further management should be provided to the women. The fFN swab is taken prior to the transvaginal scan because manipulation of the cervix, through vaginal examination or scan, for example, can cause a falsely elevated result.

The fFN testing procedure

The sample is taken using a fFN sample test kit and a speculum. The swab provided is rotated in the posterior vaginal fornix for 10 seconds, after which it is placed in the fluid in the collection tube. The shaft of the swab is snapped off and the lid closed (Figure 4.4).

The manufacturer (Hologic Inc.) recommends not using lubricating gel. This is due to a theoretical possibility that the sample may be diluted by the gel and give an inaccurately low result. However, placing a speculum without lubricating gel can be difficult and uncomfortable. An audit carried out in a busy specialist preterm clinic, comparing fFN test results when swabs were taken with and without gel (857 tests), concluded that any differences were too small to be of clinical

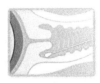 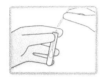 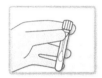

rotate swab across posterior fornix for 10 seconds

insert swab into tube and break

align swab with cap and seal tube

Figure 4.4 How to take a fetal fibronectin test swab

Source: Image from Hologic video 'Collecting a fFN specimen' YouTube: https://youtu.be/uo9x7sEhr_Q?si=L3q0YNCyx6ZB1BSS

significance (Fligelstone *et al.*, 2022) and some clinics therefore continue to use lubricating gel when carrying out fFN testing.

The presence of blood or semen (sexual intercourse within the last 48 hours) in a fFN sample can sometimes lead to a falsely elevated, or invalid, result. However, low readings are still valid and can be used to direct care as per local guidelines; some units use a threshold of 50ng/ml or 200ng/ml, while others are guided by the result of the QUiPP App, as explained below.

Processing the fFN test in the analyser

Training should be provided for those processing the sample in the point-of-care test analyser, however, a summary of the steps involved is listed below:

1   Select 'Test patient'.
2   Enter user (person running the test) initials.
3   Enter patient identifier (name or hospital number).
4   Enter Cassette Lot (batch number of test cartridge, analyser will have been calibrated to each batch).
5   Place cartridge in slot and press 'Next'
6   Wait while the analyser checks the cartridge.
7   When instructed, pipette 200 mcl of fluid (using fFN-specific pipette or Gilsen pipette)
8   Press 'Next' to start the test.

When the test is complete, the result will appear in the window and a label will be printed. The result and its implications should be explained to the woman and documented in her maternity record.

Screening for vaginal and urinary tract infections

Whether asymptomatic screening for vaginal and urinary tract infections is part of the specialist preterm service will depend on local policies, which vary between hospitals. There has long been an association between urinary tract infection and increased risk of preterm birth (Werter *et al.*, 2021), and testing is frequently offered to those attending specialist preterm monitoring (Carlisle *et al.*, 2023). This may be part of routine surveillance or when women report symptoms. Some vaginal infections, and bacterial vaginosis (BV), have also been associated with an increased risk of preterm birth. If suspected, they should be tested and treated if a positive result is returned. For more details on infection and its association with preterm birth, see Chapter 2: Causes of spontaneous preterm birth.

Planning the next steps

At the end of the appointment an explanation of findings should be provided, along with their implications, and any interventions that may be recommended. The next appointment, or discharge if appropriate, should also be arranged. These management decisions can be supported by clinical decision support tools, such as the QUiPP App. This is a validated MHRA-registered medical device which has been developed to provide fast and accessible risk assessment for women at risk of preterm birth (Carter *et al.*, 2020; Watson *et al.*, 2020). This widely used, straightforward mobile app combines risk factors and test results to calculate a simple individualised percentage risk of delivery. Risk factors, gestation at testing, cervical length and/or fetal fibronectin results are entered, and the likelihood of spontaneous preterm birth at various clinically important time points is displayed. The device can be used for asymptomatic women with known risk factors of preterm birth, as shown in Figure 4.5, or for women with or without known risk factors

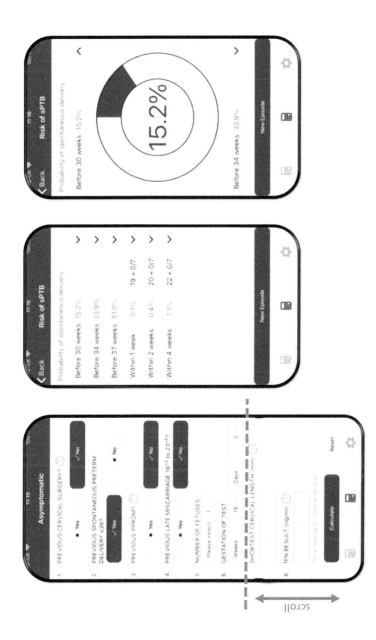

Figure 4.5 Screenshots of the QUiPP App clinical decision support tool

who are experiencing symptoms of threatened preterm labour. The app is available free of charge online (quipp.org) and as a downloadable mobile app for use on Apple (iPhone) and Android devices.

Whether another appointment, or discharge from the clinic, is planned, the woman should be advised that if she experiences pain or tightenings, unusual vaginal discharge or any other concerns, she should not hesitate to call her hospital or come in for assessment, at whichever unit is appropriate for her gestation according to local protocols, e.g. early pregnancy unit, triage, maternity assessment unit or labour ward. It is important to check she is in possession of the correct contact numbers. It may be helpful to advise the woman to inform the department at the point of calling that she is under the preterm birth surveillance team, so that her call can be triaged appropriately.

Record keeping

Hospitals, and specialist clinics within them, will have their own systems for maternity record keeping, be that paper, electronic or combination of both. Whatever overall system is used, an additional paper record, or electronic episode, may be useful to capture more detailed information relevant to preterm care. See Figure 4.6 for an example of a double-sided A4 specialist preterm clinic record sheet. This could be adapted to capture any other locally required information. If hand-held records are used, it is useful to print blank record sheets on coloured paper as this makes them easier to find quickly in the women's maternity notes.

Another resource used by an increasing number of preterm clinics is the Preterm Clinical Network (PCN) Database (www.medscinet.net/ukpcn). This is free to use and open to everyone providing specialist preterm care to women at risk, whether they are asymptomatic high-risk women or those with symptoms of threatened preterm labour or mid-trimester loss. The database can be used to store clinical data for local audit, as well as provide data that may be included in large cohort or longer term follow-up studies. Applications for data for use in these studies are subject to Research Ethics Committee and Database Access Committee approval (Carter *et al.*, 2018).

Specialist Preterm Clinic Record Sheet

Name:			Occupation:			
MRN No.: NHS No.: DOB:			Contact No: OK to leave message: Y / N Email:			
			PCN dbase consent: Yes / declined		ID.	
EDD:	G	P	Hgt		Wgt	Ethn
Country of birth			Primary language			
Intended delivery centre:		Comments:				

fFN 1

(Space for result sticker)

Risk factors/reasons for referral

Hx cervical surgery: Yes / No Type:..............Year/s........... LA / GA >1cm: Y / N / Unk

Smoking: Never / Ex ..../ Current	Other risk factors/history:
Recurrent UTI:	
Uterine anomaly:	
AQ (routine enquiry):	

fFN 2

Past Obstetric History

Year						
Gestation						
Outcome e.g. A+W, Misc, SB, NND						
PPROM						
Onset of labour						
Bleeding > 24 h						
Cervical cerclage (gest, indication & type)						
Progesterone						
Other intervention						
Mode of delivery (if CS, in-labour dilata- tion)						
Other (e.g. NND, Chorioamnionitis, SCBU)						

fFN 3

fFN 6

fFN 5

fFN 4

Figure 4.6 Example of a two-sided A4 specialist preterm clinic record sheet (front)

Source: Adapted from a record sheet used in authors' preterm clinic, with permission

Clinical Assessment

	1	2	3	4	5	6
Date (dd/mm/yy):						
Gestation (weeks)						
Mental well-being Screening question scores	PHQ8 / GAD7 /PR10 / /	PHQ8 / GAD7 /PR10 / /	PHQ8 / GAD7 /PR10 / /	PHQ8 / GAD7 /PR10 / /	PHQ8 / GAD7 /PR10 / /	PHQ8 / GAD7 /PR10 / /
Cx length 1 (mm)						
Cx length 2 (mm)						
Cx length 3 (mm)						
Funnel (mm x mm)						
Pressure Effect (Y/N)						
Length above stitch						
Sludge (Y/N)						
Sexual Int(<48hrs) (						
Douching (<48hrs)						
Placenta Praevia						
Symptoms:						
FFN result						
QUIPP % risk < 1 wk						
< 2 wks						
< 4 wks						
Plan (follow up/ discharge)						
Seen by (initials):						
Research participation:						
Swabs /Bloods—Y/N						
Other comments						

Interventions this pregnancy (related to PTB) e.g. cerclage, progesterone, admission, steroids, bedrest etc.

Intervention	Sub-type	Indication	Date	Gestation

Research recruitment criteria:	Outcome	Comments
[Research project] Eligibility criteria: [########; #######]	Date of Del: Gest: PPROM? Y / N Date: Onset of labour ?: Mode of Del: Outcome:-	

Figure 4.6 Example of a two-sided A4 specialist preterm clinic record sheet (back)

Summary

This chapter details the care that may be provided to high-risk women when they attend a specialist preterm surveillance clinic. This may help midwives to prepare women in their care in advance or to explain why certain procedures have been offered if she later asks. It may also help midwives interested in taking on a specialist role or working in these specialist clinics.

Box 4.2 **Chapter summary and recommendations for practice**

- Midwives with an understanding of specialist preterm care can support women before, during and after their appointments at the specialist preterm clinic.
- An initial assessment should start with a comprehensive history taking, with a focus on factors that affect the risk of preterm birth.
- Specialist preterm clinic monitoring usually involves transvaginal ultrasound scans for measurement of cervical length, but can also include fetal fibronectin testing, and screening for vaginal and urinary tract infections.
- Clinical decision support tools, such as the QUiPP App, can help guide management by providing individualised risk prediction.

References

Abbott, D. S., Radford, S. K., Seed, P. T., Tribe, R. M., & Shennan, A. H. 2013. Evaluation of a quantitative fetal fibronectin test for spontaneous preterm birth in symptomatic women. *American Journal of Obstetrics and Gynecology*, *208*(2), 122.e1–122.e6. https://doi.org/10.1159/000314018

Banerjee, A., Al-Dabbach, Z., Bredaki, F. E., Casagrandi, D., Tetteh, A., Greenwold, N., Ivan, M., Jurkovic, D., David, A. L., & Napolitano, R. 2022. Reproducibility of assessment of full-dilatation Cesarean section scar in women undergoing second-trimester screening for preterm birth. *Ultrasound in Obstetrics & Gynecology*, *60*(3), 396–403. https://doi.org/10.1159/000314018

Boyd, E., & Heritage, J. 2006. Taking the history: Questioning during comprehensive history-taking. *Studies in Interactional Sociolinguistics*, *20*, 151.

Carlisle, N., Care, A., Anumba, D. O., Dalkin, S., Sandall, J., & Shennan, A. H. 2023. How are hospitals in England caring for women at risk of preterm birth in 2021? The influence of national guidance on preterm birth care in England: A national questionnaire. *BMC Pregnancy and Childbirth*, *23*(1), 47. https://doi.org/10.1159/000314018

Carter, J., Seed, P. T., Watson, H. A., David, A. L., Sandall, J., Shennan, A. H., & Tribe, R. M. 2020. Development and validation of predictive models for QUiPP App v. 2: Tool for predicting preterm birth in women with symptoms of threatened preterm labor. *Ultrasound in Obstetrics & Gynecology*, 55(3), 357–367. https://doi.org/10.1159/000314018

Carter, J., Tribe, R. M., Sandall, J., and Shennan, A.H. 2018. The Preterm Clinical Network (PCN) Database: A web-based systematic method of collecting data on the care of women at risk of preterm birth. *BMC Pregnancy and Childbirth*, 18, 1–9.

Fligelstone, H., Shennan, A. H., & Carlisle, N. 2022. Does the use of lubricating gel on the speculum during fetal fibronectin testing affect the result? An audit from a larger inner-city preterm birth surveillance clinic. *Midwives Midwifery Digest (MIDIRS)*, 32(3), 357. https://doi.org/10.1159/000314018

Foster, C., & Shennan, A. H. 2014. Fetal fibronectin as a biomarker of preterm labor: A review of the literature and advances in its clinical use. *Biomarkers in Medicine*, 8(4), 471–484. https://doi.org/10.1159/000314018

Honest, H., Bachmann, L. M., Coomarasamy, A., Gupta, J. K., Kleijnen, J., & Khan, K. S. 2002. Accuracy of cervical transvaginal sonography in predicting preterm birth: A systematic review. *Ultrasound in Obstetrics & Gynecology*, 22(3), 305–322. https://doi.org/10.1159/000314018

Kroenke, K., Spitzer, R. L., & Williams, J. B. 2001. The PHQ-9: Validity of a brief depression severity measure. *Journal of General Internal Medicine*, 16(9), 606–613. https://doi.org/10.1159/000314018

Leitich, H., Egarter, C., Kaider, A., Hohlagschwandtner, M., Berghammer, P., & Husslein, P. 1999. Cervicovaginal fetal fibronectin as A marker for preterm delivery: A meta-analysis. *American Journal of Obstetrics and Gynecology*, 180(5), 1169–1176. https://doi.org/10.1159/000314018

Lockwood, C. J., Senyei, A. E., Dische, M. R., Casal, D., Shah, K. D., Thung, S. N., Jones, L., Deligdisgh, L., & Garite, T. J. 1991. Fetal fibronectin in cervical and vaginal secretions as a predictor of preterm delivery. *New England Journal of Medicine*, 325(10), 669–674. https://doi.org/10.1159/000314018

Matsuura, H., Takio, K., Titani, K., Greene, T., Levery, S. B., Salyan, M. E., & Hakomori, S. 1988. The oncofetal structure of human fibronectin defined by monoclonal antibody FDC-6. Unique structural requirement for the antigenic specificity provided by a glycosylhexapeptide. *The Journal of Biological Chemistry*, 263(7), 3314–3322. https://doi.org/10.1159/000314018

National Institute for Health and Care Excellence (NICE) (2015). Preterm Labour and Birth. NICE guideline. Last updated June 2022. Available online: https://www.nice.org.uk/guidance/ng25 Accessed: 20/04/2024

Peaceman, A. M., Andrews, W. W., Thorp, J. M., Cliver, S. P., Lukes, A., Iams, J. D., Coultrip, L., Eriksen, N., Holbrook, R. H., Elliott, J., Ingardia, C., &

Pietrantoni, M. 1997. Fetal fibronectin as a predictor of preterm birth in patients with symptoms: A multicenter trial. *American Journal of Obstetrics and Gynecology*, *177*(1), 13–18. https://doi.org/10.1159/000314018

Spitzer, R. L., Kroenke, K., Williams, J. B., & Löwe, B. 2006 May 22. A brief measure for assessing generalized anxiety disorder: The GAD-7. *Archives of Internal Medicine*. *166*(10):1092–1097. doi: 10.1001/archinte.166.10.1092. PMID: 16717171.

Suff, N., Webley, E., Hall, M., Tribe, R. M., & Shennan, A. H. 2023. Amniotic fluid sludge is associated with earlier preterm delivery and raised cervicovaginal interleukin 8 concentrations. *American Journal of Obstetrics & Gynecology MFM*, *5*(11), 101161. https://doi.org/10.1159/000314018

Watson, H. A., Seed, P. T., Carter, J., Hezelgrave, N. L., Kuhrt, K., Tribe, R. M., & Shennan, A. H. 2020. Development and validation of predictive models for QUiPP App v. 2: Tool for predicting preterm birth in asymptomatic high-risk women. *Ultrasound in Obstetrics & Gynecology*, *55*(3), 348–356. https://doi.org/10.1159/000314018

Werter, D. E., Kazemier, B. M., Schneeberger, C., Mol, B. W., de Groot, C. J., Geerlings, S. E., & Pajkrt, E. 2021. Risk indicators for urinary tract infections in low risk pregnancy and the subsequent risk of preterm birth. *Antibiotics*, *10*(9), 1055. https://doi.org/10.1159/000314018

Chapter 5

Interventions to prevent spontaneous preterm birth

Introduction

In this chapter, interventions designed to prevent preterm birth are discussed. Although the body of evidence behind these interventions is growing, it remains limited and as a result, practice varies considerably (Carlisle *et al.*, 2023). These interventions are: progesterone supplementation, cerclage (cervical suture or stitch), cervical pessary, bedrest and other restrictions of activities. Until we understand more about the mechanisms that cause preterm labour (see Chapter 2: Causes of spontaneous preterm birth) we will struggle to improve outcomes further, regardless of the interventions that are currently available.

Progesterone supplementation

Progesterone supplementation is one of the more common interventions used to reduce the risk of spontaneous preterm birth in high-risk women. This is because supplementing progestogens (natural or synthetic steroid hormones that bind to and activate the progesterone receptors) are thought to prevent the decline in progesterone which may play a role in the activation of labour (see Chapter 2: Causes of spontaneous preterm birth). There are two types of progesterone: natural progesterone (comparable to what the body produces, and often administered as a vaginal or rectal gel or pessary), and semi-synthetic

DOI: 10.4324/9781003380504-5

progestogens which are not commonly used in the UK. These have a different chemical structure to natural progesterone and include 17-hydroxyprogesterone caproate, which is administered as a weekly intramuscular injection (Shennan *et al.*, 2021b).

After years of contradictory evidence, the Evaluating Progestogens for Prevention of Preterm Birth International Collaborative (EPPPIC) individual patient data (IPD) analysis (Stewart *et al.*, 2021) provided some clarity. This influenced the International Federation of Gynecology and Obstetrics (FIGO) guidelines on the use of progestogens for the prevention of preterm birth. These guidelines (Shennan *et al.*, 2021b) recommend that progesterone (daily vaginal progesterone or weekly 17- hydroxyprogesterone caproate) should be offered to women with either a previous spontaneous preterm birth and/or short cervix on ultrasound scan who are pregnant with a single baby. This concurs with other guidance and reviews (Care *et al.*, 2022; National Institute for Health and Care Excellence [NICE], 2015). Progesterone is not recommended for women who are at risk of preterm birth for other reasons, e.g. multiple pregnancies, or those with a history of cervical surgery, if their cervix is a normal length and they have not had a preterm birth or mid-trimester loss (Shennan *et al.*, 2021b). For those with a multiple pregnancy and a known risk factor (e.g. previous preterm birth), the effect of progesterone is unknown (Shennan *et al.*, 2021b).

In the UK, NICE guidance recommends that progesterone (or cerclage) ***should be offered*** to women who have a history of spontaneous preterm birth (before 34 weeks) *and* a short cervix (25 mm or less), and that it ***should be considered*** in women with a history of spontaneous preterm birth (before 34 weeks) *or* a short cervix (25 mm or less). If it is prescribed, it should be started at between 16 and 24 weeks' gestation and continued until at least 34 weeks' gestation (NICE, 2015).

Women are often concerned about the potential detrimental effects of any medicine taken during pregnancy, and they can be reassured that there is currently no evidence of neurological or developmental harm in babies exposed to this progesterone supplementation as fetuses (Shennan *et al.*, 2021b). That said, the follow-up of children who were exposed to progesterone supplementation *in utero* does not yet extend into adulthood and their own experience of parenthood.

Cerclage

A cervical cerclage (suture or stitch) is an operation where a stitch is placed around the cervix with the aim to reduce preterm dilatation (Shennan et al., 2022). There are different procedures and methods of placement (low vaginal, high vaginal and transabdominal cerclage) and different reasons (indications) for their placement. Cerclages may be offered, early in pregnancy, to women with previous preterm birth or mid-trimester loss. These are known as 'history indicated' and are usually placed towards the end of the first trimester (before 14 weeks' gestation). Ultrasound-indicated cerclages are those where a short cervix has been identified on transvaginal ultrasound scan before 24 weeks. Emergency (sometimes called 'rescue') cerclages may be offered, up to 27 weeks, when the cervix has started to open and the membranes are exposed (Shennan et al., 2021a).

Cerclages are often described according to where they are placed by the obstetrician. A low vaginal cerclage (or McDonald's, after the doctor who described it in the 1950s) is the simplest procedure where the suture material is sewn into and around the cervix and tied in purse-string fashion. Each stitch is known as a 'bite', which should not cut through into the cervical os. The clinician will also note where the stitch is tied to aid removal if the woman goes into labour early, or when she reaches 37 weeks' gestation. The clinician will attempt to place it as high as possible but is restricted to the height at which the vaginal wall meets cervical tissue. In a high vaginal cerclage (or Shirodkar, after an obstetrician who developed the technique), the cerclage can be placed higher because an incision is made at the top of the vaginal wall, between the cervix and the bladder. Shirodkar/high vaginal cerclages are more difficult to remove as the process is more complex. Some believe that a high vaginal cerclage is more effective than a low vaginal cerclage, although evidence does not always support this. In the MAVRIC trial, which compared transabdominal cerclage with low and high vaginal cerclages in women with previous failed vaginal cerclage, high vaginal cerclage was no more effective than low vaginal cerclage in preventing preterm birth (Shennan et al., 2020).

A transabdominal cerclage (also known as a TAC) is placed as high as it is possible, at the top of the cervix, which can only be accessed through the abdominal wall. The procedure can be undertaken either by laparotomy (open surgery) or laparoscopy (key-hole surgery) (Tulandi *et al.*, 2014), although there is currently no evidence to support a favoured technique or timing. Surgeons prefer to site a transabdominal cerclage prior to pregnancy due to the lower anaesthetic risks and the technical advantages of undertaking surgery on a non-gravid uterus (Shennan *et al.*, 2021a). Neither fertility nor management of early miscarriage is impacted by transabdominal cerclage (Shennan *et al.*, 2021a). However, an *in utero* fetal death at later gestations may result in the need for a hysterotomy (an incision made in the uterus). Birth after transabdominal cerclage is usually by elective caesarean section (Carlisle *et al.*, 2017), and it can be left in place to support further pregnancies, or removed at caesarean if the woman has completed her family. The placement positions of the different cerclages are shown in Figure 5.1.

The choice of cerclage depends on the woman's history and current gestation, and clinician preference, but it is not always clear which method would be most suitable, or effective, in each case (Pilarski *et al.*, 2024). Some clinicians are more experienced and confident in placing high vaginal cerclages than their colleagues, while others do not feel the evidence is strong enough to ever offer emergency cerclages. The choice of cerclage material and insertion can also be at the surgeon's discretion (Hodgetts Morton *et al.*, 2022; Shennan *et al.*, 2021a). A woman who has had a failed vaginal cerclage in a previous pregnancy may be offered a transabdominal cerclage, and although placement before pregnancy is preferable, some doctors may still be willing to perform this procedure if the woman is under 14 weeks' gestation.

Current clinical guidelines

In the UK, cerclage is recommended by NICE as an alternative to progesterone: it should be *offered* to women with a history of spontaneous preterm birth (before 34 weeks) *and* a short cervix (25 mm or less), and it should be *considered* in women with a history of spontaneous preterm birth (before 34 weeks) *or* a short cervix (25 mm or less) (NICE, 2015).

The International Federation of Gynecology and Obstetrics (FIGO) guidelines (Shennan *et al.*, 2021a) recommend that women who have had three or more preterm deliveries and/or mid-trimester losses should be offered a history-indicated cerclage, and that ultrasound-indicated cerclage should be offered to women with a short cervix (<25 mm) and experience of one or more spontaneous preterm birth and/or mid-trimester losses. Research suggests ultrasound-indicated cerclage does not show any benefit in women with a short cervix and risk factors other than previous preterm birth or mid-trimester loss. There is an absence of strong evidence to support either ultrasound- or history-indicated cerclage in women carrying a multiple pregnancy without additional risk factors. However, if cerclage is being considered in women carrying twins, FIGO suggests that it is more likely to benefit those with a shorter cervix (less than 15 mm) (Shennan *et al.*, 2021a). FIGO highlights that neither ultrasound- nor history-indicated vaginal cerclage insertion is associated with an increased risk of preterm prelabour rupture of membranes (PPROM), chorioamnionitis, or caesarean section (Shennan *et al.*, 2021a). When women present with exposed membranes, FIGO guidelines state that an emergency cerclage may be considered, but counselling should include an increased risk of infection to both mother and baby in these circumstances (Shennan *et al.*, 2021a).

FIGO recommends that a transabdominal cerclage should be recommended to women who have previously had a failed transvaginal cerclage, i.e. a preterm birth or mid-trimester loss before 28 weeks' gestation after an ultrasound- or history-indicated cerclage (not an emergency or 'rescue' cerclage) (Shennan *et al.*, 2021a). This is based on evidence from the MAVRIC trial, in which women randomised to the transabdominal cerclage group were much less likely to have a preterm birth compared to women randomised to low or high vaginal cerclage (Shennan *et al.*, 2020).

Cerclage removal

Transabdominal cerclages can be left *in-situ* to support subsequent pregnancies, while vaginally placed cerclages are removed at around

37 weeks unless labour starts earlier. Low vaginal cerclages can usually be removed in a labour ward room without anaesthesia, although Entonox may be offered if the woman is very uncomfortable. High vaginal cerclages require removal in theatre under spinal anaesthetic.

Box 5.1 In her own words: woman's experience of transabdominal cerclage

'Following my second preterm loss, at just under 18 weeks, I researched online what my options would be should we decide to try to become pregnant again. The TAC and TVC were what I found, The TVC seemed to be the most common method, the TAC seemed like it was only an option if the TVC failed previously or as a last resort.

I asked my GP to be referred to a clinic in my area which had a specialist preterm prevention clinic and I waited a few weeks for an appointment to come through. At the appointment I was recommended a history-indicated TVC at approximately 12 weeks.

Luckily, we fell pregnant quickly and when I reached 12 weeks I was admitted to hospital for the procedure. Unfortunately, my waters still "went", and my son was born at 23 weeks. He survived 9 weeks in NICU. Some weeks following his death I received a call from my consultant who had "just been informed of Harry's passing", so she immediately called to offer her condolences. She asked if my husband and I would like an appointment to see her to discuss our options should we want to try for another baby.

At the appointment she provided us with in-depth information about the TAC in general, its benefits, the procedure, how it differs from a TVC. I came out of the appointment feeling very well informed. The procedure was scheduled in for 6 weeks' time. I was very sceptical before the procedure as I had put my entire faith into the TVC and it had failed; what was going to make this time any different?

I was met on the day of surgery by my consultant and another who had been brought in from a neighbouring hospital. They reassured me and explained how long the procedure would take, how long I would be asleep etc. I wish I had been told about the swelling of my tummy beforehand. I woke up with a swollen tummy which was very triggering for me following as it instantly reminded me of being pregnant. I also hadn't been told at any point before the day of my pre-op, that the procedure would require me to be put to sleep; I had assumed it would be a spinal injection and I would be awake, just as the TVC had been.

The anxiety of my waters going in my previous pregnancy never left me during my TAC pregnancy; I found it very difficult to "believe" the TAC would work when the TVC had failed. I had milestones in my head: 21 weeks when my waters broke; 23 weeks when I delivered Harry; 27 weeks a doctor told the lady in the bed opposite me when I had Harry that at 27 weeks a baby's chances of survival in NICU are very good…and with each passing one of those it did get a little easier.

My consultant was excellent, she had me in the hospital every 3 weeks for scans to check my TAC from 12 to 27 weeks. It never changed, it kept my baby safe inside and my consultant delivered him into my arms at 37 weeks exactly. I found it so beneficial having the same consultant see me at each appointment, and to deliver my son also.'

Claire G

Cervical (Arabin or vaginal) pessary

Another, currently less common (at least in the UK) intervention to prevent preterm birth is a cervical pessary (sometimes called a vaginal pessary, or an Arabin pessary, after the gynaecologist who developed it in the 1970s). This is a device composed of synthetic material which is placed in the vagina and around the cervix (Figure 5.1). The pessary adjusts the angle of the cervix to be more posterior which, it is hypothesised, reduces pressure on it and therefore prevents cervical shortening and preterm labour.

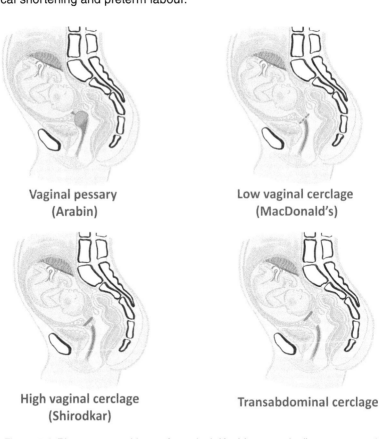

Vaginal pessary
(Arabin)

Low vaginal cerclage
(MacDonald's)

High vaginal cerclage
(Shirodkar)

Transabdominal cerclage

Figure 5.1 Placement positions of cervical (Arabin or vaginal) pessary, and vaginal and transabdominal cerclages

Artist: Gemma Baxter

How, physiologically, a more posterior cervix makes preterm birth less likely has yet to be explained, and FIGO considers that there is not enough evidence to promote the use of cervical pessaries as a standard treatment for reducing preterm birth rates (Grobman et al., 2021). A 2022 Cochrane review concluded that pessaries may decrease preterm birth in women with singleton pregnancy compared to no treatment or vaginal progesterone; however, the evidence advocating this was not robust (Abdel-Aleem *et al.*, 2022).

Bedrest and avoidance of activity

For many years, bedrest and avoidance of activity, including sex, have been recommended to women at risk of preterm birth. There is, however, no evidence that bedrest at home or within a hospital prevents preterm labour or birth (Sosa *et al.*, 2015). Despite this, it is often still recommended, even though there are risks associated with it, such as blood clots from immobility, weight gain, poor mental health and anxiety and other detrimental effects of being away from family and support network if the woman has been hospitalised. These factors need to be considered carefully and discussed with the woman during care planning (Sosa *et al.*, 2015). Sexual intercourse and physical exercise are all possible with any of the cerclages or the cervical (Arabin or vaginal) pessary in place. Some clinicians will advise limiting physical activities, such as high-impact exercise and sexual intercourse, whilst not advocating strict bedrest. If a woman decides herself to substantially limit her physical activity, a prescription of prophylactic anticoagulant medication may be considered appropriate.

Evidence (what little there is) around the restriction of activity in pregnancy is unclear, largely because it includes women who are at high risk of preterm birth for a mixture of reasons (e.g. some with previous preterm birth, some with short cervical length, some with and some without symptoms). One study found that in asymptomatic women with a short cervix (<30 mm) but no history of preterm birth, undertaking exercise and sexual intercourse was actually associated with a *reduced* risk of preterm birth (Saccone *et al.*, 2018). Another found that restricting activity (of any type) did not reduce preterm birth in asymptomatic nulliparous women with a short cervix ≤ 25 mm (Grobman et al., 2013). This may be due to the beneficial effects on reducing anxiety and stress that exercise provides women, alongside additional closeness to their partner (Goodfellow *et al.*, 2021). Therefore, for asymptomatic women with a short cervix and without a history of a prior spontaneous preterm birth, the advice of avoiding sexual intercourse could be seen as overcautious.

In Goodfellow *et al.*'s (2021) review of the evidence, no research regarding sexual intercourse and women with a short cervix and a history of previous spontaneous preterm birth could be found. Some clinicians would therefore recommend restricting sexual intercourse due to the absence of data (MacPhedran, 2018). Meanwhile, others feel it is important to recognise the benefits of intimacy on the woman's wellbeing and would offer prudent advice such as only limiting sex when the cervix is especially short, e.g. below 15 mm (Goodfellow *et al.*, 2021). Other clinicians may disagree and be comfortable with a higher or lower threshold.

Where a woman has preterm prelabour rupture of membranes (PPROM), the consensus appears to be to advise avoiding sexual activity (Goodfellow *et al.*, 2021). Evidence has demonstrated a relationship between the time of the first vaginal examination following the rupture of membranes and delivery or maternal infection (Lewis *et al.*, 1992). In the same way that clinicians try to limit vaginal examinations in women who have ruptured their membranes, it is reasonable to advise women to avoid penetrative sexual activity if their membranes have ruptured. This is because penetrative sexual activity could provide the same mechanism to trigger labour (presumably of ascending infection) (Goodfellow *et al.*, 2021).

In summary, there is a lack of evidence regarding bedrest and avoidance of activity and this should be discussed with women at high risk of preterm birth, along with the pros and cons of both avoiding and continuing activity. Lack of evidence does not equate to proof of harm or safety, and avoiding activity brings its own potential dangers. Nuanced conversations, exploring what is most important to the individual woman should support her in making informed decisions.

Summary

The most common interventions to prevent preterm birth are described in this chapter. This knowledge will help midwives answer questions from women in their care who may have been offered or already received them. If the midwife or woman needs further information they should not hesitate to contact their local preterm team for clarification.

Box 5.2 **Chapter summary and recommendations for practice**

- Progesterone supplementation, cerclages and cervical (Arabin or vaginal) pessaries are interventions which may be offered when a woman is at high risk of preterm birth.
- Cerclages can be inserted vaginally or transabdominally.
- There is no evidence that bedrest prevents preterm birth or preterm labour.
- There is a lack of evidence regarding avoidance of activity (such as sexual intercourse) for women at risk of preterm birth.

References

Abdel-Aleem, H., Shaaban, O. M., Abdel-Aleem, M. A., & Aboelfadle Mohamed, A. 2022. Cervical pessary for preventing preterm birth in singleton pregnancies. *Cochrane Database of Systematic Reviews*, *12*. https://doi.org/10.1002/14651858.CD014508

Care, A., Nevitt, S. J., Medley, N., Donegan, S., Good, L., Hampson, L., Tudur Smith, C., & Alfirevic, Z. 2022. Interventions to prevent spontaneous preterm birth in women with singleton pregnancy who are at high risk: Systematic review and network meta-analysis. *BMJ*, *376*, e064547. https://doi.org/10.1136/bmj-2021-064547

Carlisle, N., Ridout, A. E., & Shennan, A. H. 2017. Successful vaginal delivery following an abdominal cerclage removal in pre-term labour. *International Journal of Obstetrics and Gynaecology Study*, *1*(1).

Carlisle, N., Care, A., Anumba, D. O., Dalkin, S., Sandall, J., & Shennan, A. H. 2023. How are hospitals in England caring for women at risk of preterm birth in 2021? The influence of national guidance on preterm birth care in England: A national questionnaire. *BMC Pregnancy and Childbirth*, *23*(1), 47. https://doi.org/10.1159/000314018

Goodfellow, L., Care, A., & Alfirevic, Z. 2021. Controversies in the prevention of spontaneous preterm birth in asymptomatic women: An evidence summary and expert opinion. *BJOG: An International Journal of Obstetrics & Gynaecology*, *128*(2), 177–194. https://doi.org/10.1111/1471-0528.16544

Grobman, W. A., Gilbert, S. A., Iams, J. D., Spong, C. Y., Saade, G., Mercer, B. M., Tita, A. T. N., Rouse, D. J., Sorokin, Y., Leveno, K. J., Tolosa, J. E., Thorp, J. M., Caritis, S. N., & Peter Van Dorsten, J., & Network*, for the E. K. S. N. I. of C. H. and H. D. (NICHD) M.-F. M. U. (MFMU). 2013. Activity restriction among women with a short cervix. *Obstetrics & Gynecology*, *121*(6). https://journals.lww.com/greenjournal/Fulltext/2013/06000/Activity_Restriction_Among_Women_With_a_Short.7.aspx

Grobman, W. A., Norman, J., & Jacobsson, B., & Birth, the F. W. G. for P. 2021. FIGO good practice recommendations on the use of pessary for reducing the frequency and improving outcomes of preterm birth. *International Journal of Gynecology & Obstetrics*, *155*(1), 23–25. https://doi.org/10.1002/ijgo.13837

Hodgetts Morton, V., Toozs-Hobson, P., Moakes, C. A., Middleton, L., Daniels, J., Simpson, N. A. B., Shennan, A., Israfil-Bayli, F., Ewer, A. K., Gray, J., Slack, M., Norman, J. E., Lees, C., Tryposkiadis, K., Hughes, M., Brocklehurst, P., & Morris, R. K. 2022. Monofilament suture versus braided suture thread to improve pregnancy outcomes after vaginal cervical cerclage (c-STICH): A pragmatic randomised, controlled, phase 3, superiority trial. *The Lancet*, *400*(10361), 1426–1436. https://doi.org/10.1016/S0140-6736(22)01808-6

Lewis, D., Major, C., Towers, C., Asrat, T., Harding, J., & Garite, T. 1992. Effects of digital vaginal examinations on latency period in preterm premature rupture of membranes. *Obstetrics & Gynecology*, *80*, 630–634.

MacPhedran, S. E. 2018. Sexual activity recommendations in high-risk pregnancies: What is the evidence? *Sexual Medicine Reviews*, *6*(3), 343–357. https://doi.org/10.1016/j.sxmr.2018.01.004

National Institute for Health and Care Excellence (NICE). 2015. Preterm Labour and Birth. NICE guideline. Last updated June 2022. Available online: https://www.nice.org.uk/guidance/ng25 Accessed: 20/04/2024

Pilarski, N., Morris, R. K., & Hodgetts-Morton, V., 2024. Does a stitch in time save lives? An update on the evidence for cervical cerclage in 2024. *Obstetrics, Gynaecology & Reproductive Medicine*, *34*(6), 167–170.

Saccone, G., Maruotti, G., Martinelli, P., & Berghella, V. 2018. 661: Exercise and sex in women with short cervix: A secondary analysis of a randomized trial. *American Journal of Obstetrics & Gynecology*, *218*(1), S396–S397. https://doi.org/10.1016/j.ajog.2017.11.191

Shennan, A., Chandiramani, M., Bennett, P., David, A. L., Girling, J., Ridout, A., Seed, P. T., Simpson, N., Thornton, S., Tydeman, G., Quenby, S., & Carter, J. 2020. MAVRIC: A multicenter randomized controlled trial of transabdominal vs transvaginal cervical cerclage. *American Journal of Obstetrics and Gynecology,222*(3),261.e1–261.e9.https://doi.org/10.1016/j.ajog.2019.09.040

Shennan, A. H., Story, L., Royal College of Obstetricians, Gynaecologists. 2022. Cervical cerclage: Green-top guideline no. 75. *BJOG: An International Journal of Obstetrics & Gynaecology, 129*(7), 1178–1210. https://doi.org/10.1159/000314018

Shennan, A., Story, L., Jacobsson, B., & Grobman, W. A., & Birth, the F. W. G. for P. 2021a. FIGO good practice recommendations on cervical cerclage for prevention of preterm birth. *International Journal of Gynecology & Obstetrics, 155*(1), 19–22. https://doi.org/10.1002/ijgo.13835

Shennan, A., Suff, N., Leigh Simpson, J., Jacobsson, B., Mol, B. W., & Grobman, W. A., & Birth, the F. W. G. for P. 2021b. FIGO good practice recommendations on progestogens for prevention of preterm delivery. *International Journal of Gynecology & Obstetrics, 155*(1), 16–18. https://doi.org/10.1002/ijgo.13852

Sosa, C. G., Althabe, F., Belizán, J. M., & Bergel, E. 2015. Bed rest in singleton pregnancies for preventing preterm birth. *Cochrane Database of Systematic Reviews, 3*. https://doi.org/10.1002/14651858.CD003581.pub3

Stewart, L. A., Simmonds, M., Duley, L., Llewellyn, A., Sharif, S., Walker, R. A. E., Beresford, L., Wright, K., Aboulghar, M. M., Alfirevic, Z., Azargoon, A., Bagga, R., Bahrami, E., Blackwell, S. C., Caritis, S. N., Combs, C. A., Croswell, J. M., Crowther, C. A., Das, A. F., …, & Walley, T. 2021. Evaluating progestogens for preventing preterm birth international collaborative (EPPPIC): Meta-analysis of individual participant data from randomised controlled trials. *The Lancet, 397*(10280), 1183–1194. https://doi.org/10.1016/S0140-6736(21)00217-8

Tulandi, T., Alghanaim, N., Hakeem, G., & Tan, X. 2014. Pre and post-conceptional abdominal cerclage by laparoscopy or laparotomy. *Journal of Minimally Invasive Gynecology, 21*(6), 987–993. https://doi.org/10.1016/j.jmig.2014.05.015

Chapter 6
Interventions to improve neonatal outcomes

Introduction

This chapter outlines the interventions that are designed to reduce the neonatal mortality and morbidities associated with preterm birth when it cannot be prevented. These interventions include antenatal corticosteroids (steroids), magnesium sulphate, tocolysis, antibiotics, admission to hospital and *in utero* transfer.

Perinatal optimisation

The British Association of Perinatal Medicine's 'Perinatal Optimisation Care Pathway' (BAPM, 2020) offers guidance to optimising the care of preterm babies in order to give them the best possible start in life, and to reduce their chance of death and short- and long-term morbidities (Figure 6.1). The elements 'Prediction of preterm birth' are covered in Chapter 4: Specialist care for the woman at risk and Chapter 7: Care of the woman in threatened preterm labour. In this chapter, the elements within the 'Antenatal Optimisation' and 'Peripartum Optimisation' are discussed below.

Place of birth

Babies born preterm have better outcomes if they are delivered at a hospital with an appropriate neonatal unit level for that baby (Lasswell *et al.*, 2010; Lee *et al.*, 2003; Marlow *et al.*, 2014; Zeitlin *et al.*, 2016).

DOI: 10.4324/9781003380504-6

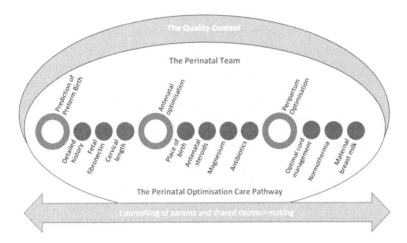

Figure 6.1 British Association of Perinatal Medicine 'Perinatal Optimisation Care Pathway'

Source: BAPM (2020)

The optimum place for a preterm baby to be born depends on its gestation and expected birth weight. In the UK, Level 3 neonatal units, which include neonatal intensive care, provide care for all babies at gestations after 22^{+6} weeks. Level 2 units provide care for singletons from 26^{+6} weeks gestation and twins or higher multiples from 27^{+6} weeks, providing the predicted birth weight is over 800 g. Level 1 units (also called special care baby units) typically provide care after 31^{+6} weeks, provided the predicted birth weight is above 1000 g (Watson *et al.*, 2020).

If a woman is at high risk of preterm labour, then she should be transferred to a hospital unit with the appropriate level neonatal unit. This is because babies that are born and then transferred after birth (*ex utero*) have higher rates of mortality and morbidity than those transferred *in utero* (babies whose mothers were transferred while still pregnant) (Finnström *et al.*, 1997; Helenius *et al.*, 2019; Synnes *et al.*, 2017). Predicting preterm birth is difficult, as discussed in previous chapters, but it can be aided by predictive tests (e.g. cervical length and fetal fibronectin) and clinical decision support tools, such as the QUiPP App (as explained in Chapter 4: Specialist care for the woman at risk).

In utero transfers (IUT) also prevent maternal separation from the baby which can occur when transferred *ex utero* (Watson *et al.*, 2020). However, any transfer will result in difficulties for the woman and her family, including separation from older children as well as the impact on the woman's partner (Porcellato *et al.*, 2015). Financial strain can result from travel costs to the transferred hospital, accommodation, and unpaid leave for partners (Watson *et al.*, 2020). Stress and anxiety are often associated with this difficult period, and as previously discussed, evidence shows that stress can increase adverse pregnancy outcomes (Dole *et al.*, 2003; Latendresse, 2009). The midwife's holistic assessment of women admitted to hospital, or transferred from another, should include their mental wellbeing alongside their physical needs. This is discussed in more detail in Chapter 7: Care of the woman in hospital.

Both *in utero* and *ex utero* transfers are difficult to arrange and manage. They involve communication with, and co-ordination of, midwifery, obstetric and neonatal teams at often several potentially suitable units. While there is currently no national co-ordinated approach in England, there are some local networks, working within geographical regions, which attempt to streamline this process. These include cot locating services, such as the Emergency Bed Service in London. In Scotland, a national approach includes a framework for hospitals which advises use of the QUiPP App when women present in threatened preterm labour and a dedicated *in utero* co-ordination service (ICS) called ScotSTAR (Scottish Perinatal Network Transport Group, 2023).

Antenatal corticosteroids

Administration of antenatal corticosteroids is one of the most important interventions to enhance neonatal outcomes in preterm babies. Evidence shows they reduce the incidence of neonatal respiratory distress syndrome, fetal and neonatal death and cerebroventricular haemorrhage (McGoldrick *et al.*, 2020; Stock *et al.*, 2022; World Health Organization, 2022).

The Royal College of Obstetricians and Gynaecologists (RCOG) recommends that corticosteroids should be offered to women between 24^{+0} and 34^{+6} weeks' gestation when imminent preterm birth is anticipated (either due to established preterm labour, preterm prelabour rupture of membranes [PPROM] or planned preterm birth) (Stock *et al.*, 2022), in both singleton and multiple pregnancies (World Health Organization, 2022). Midwives should refer to their local guidelines, but in the UK, 24 mg dexamethasone phosphate is usually given intramuscularly in two doses of 12 mg, 24 hours apart, or four doses of 6 mg, 12 hours apart (Stock *et al.*, 2022). The first dose should be given even if it is unlikely the full course will be completed because the labour is progressing quickly (World Health Organization, 2022).

The timing of antenatal corticosteroid administration is critical, as benefits are optimal when birth occurs between 24 hours and seven days after administration (World Health Organization, 2022). No benefit is seen after seven days, so if a woman is given corticosteroids but does not deliver within seven days and goes into preterm labour again later in her pregnancy, they need to be repeated.

The timing of the first course of steroids is crucial because there is increasing evidence that repeated doses could be detrimental to the fetus. Even one course of corticosteroids can result in reduced birth weight, birth length and head circumference (Rodriguez *et al.*, 2019), but babies who have been exposed to repeated courses are most affected (Crowther *et al.*, 2019).

Deciding when to offer corticosteroids is not always straightforward, because the vast majority of women with symptoms of threatened pre-term labour do not go on to deliver early. This is when clinical decision support tools such as the QUiPP App are very useful (see Chapter 4: Specialist care for the woman at risk). The British Association of Perinatal Medicine (BAPM) QUiPP App toolkit recommends hospitalisation and administration of steroids when a woman has a 5% or more chance of delivering a preterm baby within seven days (Carlisle *et al.*, 2021). This 5% threshold was chosen by a Delphi consensus of experts in preterm birth (Carter *et al.*, 2016); however, individual clinicians and/or units may have their own preferred QUiPP threshold. The RCOG concludes there is limited evidence to recommend repeated courses of corticosteroids, but if they are given, there should be no more than three courses in one preg-nancy (Stock *et al.*, 2022). The World Health Organization (WHO) recom-mends where a repeated dose is recommended, that a single dose is administered only if a woman is likely to deliver and if more than seven days have elapsed since the last course was given.

While antenatal corticosteroid therapy is recommended for women whose membranes have ruptured, it is not recommended for women with chorioamnionitis (infection of the membranes and chorion of the pla-centa) (World Health Organization, 2022). This is because corticosteroids suppress the immune system, so if a woman has a systemic infection, it is possible that her immune response could be suppressed and increase the chance of serious consequences, such as sepsis (McGoldrick *et al.*, 2020; Stock *et al.*, 2022; World Health Organization, 2022).

An additional consideration is that after administration of corticosteroids, maternal blood glucose levels rise and can remain high for up to five days (Itoh *et al.*, 2016; Jolley *et al.*, 2016). Women with diabetes should not be automatically excluded from being offered antenatal corticosteroids but, where they are given, close blood glucose monitoring according to local protocols should be undertaken, and additional insulin may be necessary (McGoldrick *et al.*, 2020; Stock *et al.*, 2022; World Health Organization, 2022).

Box 6.1 **In her own words: woman's experience of being admitted to hospital and receiving antenatal corticosteroids**

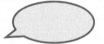

I had confirmed PPROM at 33 weeks and 1 day. I was admitted into the maternity ward immediately.

The obstetrician explained verbally and shared printed information on both PPROM and the steroid injection that evening. We were offered the injection immediately. But we declined saying we wanted a bit more time to decide. We asked about the risks and benefits and were told that it was needed to help the baby's lungs mature in case of a preterm birth. But it wasn't as effective if given more than a week before the birth.

The following morning, I was asked again if we were having the injection and I still hadn't gotten a chance to fully decide, as my husband wasn't there. We spent quite a bit of time googling, this was all so new to us. We felt like it was tricky mainly due to not knowing when the baby would be born. However, we did understand from the information given that most cases of PPROM babies are born within 7–10 days. We were so hopeful to hold onto him for longer than that, which impacted our decision making.

After discussing between ourselves, we decided to get the injection and thought the most likely outcome was that the baby would be born soon. We had the injection that day and then the next one 24 hours later, after which I was discharged. I don't remember the injection being particularly painful. It was just one of many needles I had to endure during pregnancy and delivery.

In the end we had made the right call as he was born just a few days later at 34 weeks and 1 day (within a week of the injections), and he had great Apgar scores, thankfully. We were relieved to have taken the injections when we did.

Sophia

Magnesium sulphate

Women in established preterm labour, or those having a planned preterm birth in the next 24 hours, should be offered magnesium sulphate ($MgSO_4$). This is because preterm infants have a lower chance of cerebral palsy and motor dysfunction if their mothers receive this intervention within 24 hours before their birth (Conde-Agudelo & Romero, 2009; Costantine *et al.*, 2009; Doyle *et al.*, 2009; Jung *et al.*, 2018). The benefit is greatest before 30 weeks' gestation (Costantine *et al.*, 2009), and the risk of the baby having cerebral palsy is reduced by around 30% (Doyle *et al.*, 2009).

The International Federation of Gynecology and Obstetrics (FIGO), RCOG and NICE recommend that all women giving birth before 30 weeks gestation are offered $MgSO_4$ (NICE, 2015; Shennan *et al.*, 2021; Thomson and RCOG, 2019). NICE also recommends $MgSO_4$ is considered when women are delivering between 30^{+0} and 33^{+6} weeks' gestation (NICE, 2015). FIGO similarly recommends that $MgSO_4$ is considered when women are below 34 weeks' gestation.

$MgSO_4$ should be administered when preterm birth is expected or planned within the next 24 hours, but in planned births it should be commenced as close as possible to 4 hours before the birth. If birth is planned or expected to occur within 4 hours, $MgSO_4$ may still provide some benefit, so it should be offered (Shennan *et al.*, 2021). The optimal regimen of $MgSO_4$ for fetal neuroprotection is an intravenous loading dose of 4 g (administered slowly over 20–30 minutes), followed by an hourly 1 g maintenance dose until the baby is born. It should be discontinued after 24 hours if the woman has not delivered (Shennan *et al.*, 2021).

If an *in utero* transfer is necessary, $MgSO_4$ should usually be commenced prior to transfer. The maintenance dose should then be continued until the ambulance arrives but should not be administered during the transfer. Once arrived at the destination hospital, the woman should then be assessed for recommencement of the maintenance dose.

There is no evidence of adverse neonatal outcomes following maternal administration of $MgSO_4$ (Shepherd *et al.*, 2019). However, in the mother, $MgSO_4$ generates flushing, sweating and a feeling of warmth owing to its peripheral vasodilator effects when infused intravenously. Additional maternal side effects related to dosage and speed of infusion have been reported, which include nausea, vomiting, head-ache, palpitations and, rarely, pulmonary oedema. Cardiac and neuro-logical adverse events can occur with $MgSO_4$ overdose, so women should be monitored during administration, at least four hourly, for clinical signs of magnesium toxicity (Shennan *et al.*, 2021). This involves recording maternal pulse, blood pressure, respiratory rate and deep tendon (for example patellar) reflexes.

Tocolysis

Tocolytic drugs are used to delay birth, for up to 48 hours, in women with symptoms of preterm labour. While they will not delay the birth indefi-nitely, the time gained allows administration of drugs such as antenatal corticosteroids and magnesium sulphate, and for transfer to another unit if necessary (NICE, 2015). NICE recommend that nifedipine is offered for tocolysis in women who are between 24^{+0} and 33^{+6} weeks' pregnant with intact membranes and in suspected preterm labour. Oxytocin receptor antagonists (e.g. atosiban) are recommended if nife-dipine is contraindicated.

A Cochrane review (Mackeen *et al.*, 2014) concluded that tocolysis does not significantly improve perinatal outcome and it may be associ-ated with an increased risk of chorioamnionitis. Subsequently, the RCOG does not recommend tocolysis in women whose membranes have ruptured (Thomson and RCOG, 2019).

Antibiotics

The RCOG and the BAPM Antenatal Optimisation toolkit recommend that all women who are less than 37 weeks' pregnant and in estab-lished preterm labour receive intrapartum antibiotic prophylaxis to pre-vent early onset neonatal Group B streptococcal (GBS) infection (BAPM, 2020; Hughes *et al.*, 2017). This recommendation applies to all women, regardless of whether their membranes have ruptured or not. The risk of GBS infection in babies born preterm is higher than those born at term, and the mortality rate from infection is ten times higher

(20%–30% versus 2%–3% at term) (Fairlie *et al.*, 2013; O'Sullivan *et al.*, 2015; Phares *et al.*, 2008; Schrag *et al.*, 2000). The RCOG recommend that 3 g intravenous benzylpenicillin is administered as soon as preterm labour is confirmed and then 1.5 g every 4 hours until delivery. Ideally the first dose should be given at least 4 hours prior to delivery. If the woman is allergic to penicillin, an alternative may be offered, usually cefuroxime (1.5 g loading dose followed by 750 mg every 8 hours), or intravenous vancomycin (1 g every 12 hours) (Hughes *et al.*, 2017).

Summary

In this chapter we outline the interventions that may be offered to women at imminent risk of preterm birth to reduce the chance of her baby experiencing the short- and long-term problems associated with being born too soon. Care of the baby after the birth is not within the scope of this book.

Box 6.2 **Chapter summary and recommendations for practice**

- Antenatal corticosteroids should be offered to all women (singleton or multiple pregnancies) where imminent preterm delivery is anticipated before 34^{+6} weeks' gestation. This lowers the risk of neonatal respiratory distress syndrome, fetal and neonatal death and cerebroventricular haemorrhage.
- The optimal clinical effect of antenatal corticosteroids is between 24 hours and seven days after administration, with no benefit if the woman delivers more than seven days later.
- If preterm labour recurs after seven days and birth is expected, corticosteroids may be repeated.
- Antenatal administration of corticosteroids can result in reduced birth weight, birth length and head circumference, which are more likely in babies exposed to repeated doses. This could be avoided by more accurate assessment of risk of delivery at the first episode.

- Clinical decision support tools, such as the QUiPP App, can help management decisions by providing a % chance of birth within seven days.
- $MgSO_4$ should be offered to women under 30 weeks' gestation and considered for women under 34 weeks' gestation who are expected to deliver within the next 24 hours. This lowers the risk to the baby of cerebral palsy and motor dysfunction.
- Tocolysis may be offered to women who are between 24^{+0} and 33^{+6} week's pregnant in suspected preterm labour with intact membranes to enable preparation such as administration of antenatal corticosteroids and admission or *in utero* transfer.
- All women who are less than 37 weeks' pregnant and in established preterm labour should receive intrapartum antibiotic prophylaxis to prevent early onset neonatal Group B streptococcal infection.
- Babies have better outcomes when they are born in a unit which has an appropriate neonatal unit for their gestation and clinical needs.

References

BAPM. (2020). *Antenatal Optimisation for Preterm Infants Less Than 34 Weeks, A Quality Improvement Toolkit*. Available at: https://hubble-live-assets.s3.amazonaws.com/bapm/redactor2_assets/files/843/AO_Toolkit_FULLTOOLKIT_11-2-21.docx.pdf. Accessed: 20/02/24

Carlisle, N., Watson, H. A., & Shennan, A. H. (2021). Development and rapid rollout of the QUiPP app toolkit for women who arrive in threatened preterm labour. *BMJ Open Quality*, *10*: e001272. https://doi.org/10.1136/bmjoq-2020-001272

Carter, J., Tribe, R., Watson, H., & Shennan, A. (2016). Threatened preterm labour management: Results of a Delphi consensus on best practice. *BJOG—An International Journal of Obstetrics and Gynaecology*, *123*, 100–101).

Conde-Agudelo, A., & Romero, R. (2009). Antenatal magnesium sulfate for the prevention of cerebral palsy in preterm infants less than 34 weeks' gestation:

A systematic review and metaanalysis. *American Journal of Obstetrics & Gynecology*, *200*(6), 595–609. https://doi.org/10.1016/j.ajog.2009.04.005 https://doi.org/10.1016/j.ajog.2009.04.005

Costantine, M. M., Weiner, S. J., & (MFMU), for the E. K. S. N. I. of C. H. and H. D. (NICHD) M. M. U. N. (2009). Effects of antenatal exposure to magnesium sulfate on neuroprotection and mortality in preterm infants: A meta-analysis. *Obstetrics & Gynecology*, *114*(2 Part 1). https://journals.lww.com/greenjournal/ Fulltext/2009/08000/Effects_of_Antenatal_Exposure_to_Magnesium_ Sulfate.22.aspx

Crowther, C. A., Middleton, P. F., Voysey, M., Askie, L., Zhang, S., Martlow, T. K., Aghajafari, F., Asztalos, E. V, Brocklehurst, P., Dutta, S., Garite, T. J., Guinn, D. A., Hallman, M., Hardy, P., Lee, M.-J., Maurel, K., Mazumder, P., McEvoy, C., Murphy, K. E., ... Group, the P. (2019). Effects of repeat prenatal corticosteroids given to women at risk of preterm birth: An individual participant data meta-analysis. *PLOS Medicine*, *16*(4), e1002771. https://doi.org/10.1371/ journal.pmed.1002771

Dole, N., Savitz, D. A., Hertz-Picciotto, I., Siega-Riz, A. M., McMahon, M. J., & Buekens, P. (2003). Maternal stress and preterm birth. *Obstetrical & Gynecological Survey*, *58*(6). https://journals.lww.com/obgynsurvey/Fulltext/ 2003/06000/Maternal_Stress_and_Preterm_Birth.3.aspx

Doyle, L. W., Crowther, C. A., Middleton, P., Marret, S., & Rouse, D. (2009). Magnesium sulphate for women at risk of preterm birth for neuroprotection of the fetus. *Cochrane Database of Systematic Reviews*, *1*. https://doi. org/10.1002/14651858.CD004661.pub3

Fairlie, T., Zell, E. R., & Schrag, S. (2013). Effectiveness of intrapartum antibiotic prophylaxis for prevention of early-onset group B streptococcal disease. *Obstetrics and Gynecology*, *121*(3), 570–577. https://doi.org/10.1097/ AOG.0b013e318280d4f6

Finnström, O., Olausson, P. O., Sedin, G., Serenius, F., Svenningsen, N., Thiringer, K., Tunell, R., Wennergren, M., & Wesström, G. (1997). The Swedish national prospective study on extremely low birthweight (ELBW) infants. Incidence, mortality, morbidity and survival in relation to level of care. *Acta Paediatrica*, *86*(5), 503–511. https://doi.org/10.1111/j.1651-2227.1997. tb08921.x

Helenius, K., Longford, N., Lehtonen, L., Modi, N., & Gale, C. (2019). Association of early postnatal transfer and birth outside a tertiary hospital with mortality and severe brain injury in extremely preterm infants: Observational cohort study with propensity score matching. *BMJ*, *367*. https://doi.org/10.1136/bmj. l5678

Hughes, R. G., Brocklehurst, P., Steer, P. J., & Heath, P. (2017). Stenson BM on behalf of the Royal College of Obstetricians and Gynaecologists. Prevention of early-onset neonatal group B streptococcal disease. Green-top guideline no. 36. *BJOG, 124,* e280–e305.

Itoh, A., Saisho, Y., Miyakoshi, K., Fukutake, M., Kasuga, Y., Ochiai, D., Matsumoto, T., Tanaka, M., & Itoh, H. (2016). Time-dependent changes in insulin requirement for maternal glycemic control during antenatal corticosteroid therapy in women with gestational diabetes: A retrospective study. *Endocrine Journal, 63*(1), 101–104. https://doi.org/10.1507/endocrj.EJ15-0482

Jolley, J. A., Rajan, P. V., Petersen, R., Fong, A., & Wing, D. A. (2016). Effect of antenatal betamethasone on blood glucose levels in women with and without diabetes. *Diabetes Research and Clinical Practice, 118,* 98–104. https://doi.org/10.1016/j.diabres.2016.06.005

Jung, E. J., Byun, J. M., Kim, Y. N., Lee, K. B., Sung, M. S., Kim, K. T., Shin, J. B., & Jeong, D. H. (2018). Antenatal magnesium sulfate for both tocolysis and fetal neuroprotection in premature rupture of the membranes before 32 weeks' gestation. *The Journal of Maternal-Fetal & Neonatal Medicine, 31*(11), 1431–1441. https://doi.org/10.1080/14767058.2017.1317743

Lasswell, S. M., Barfield, W. D., Rochat, R. W., & Blackmon, L. (2010). Perinatal regionalization for very low-birth-weight and very preterm infants: A meta-analysis. *JAMA, 304*(9), 992–1000. https://doi.org/10.1001/jama.2010.1226

Latendresse, G. (2009). The interaction between chronic stress and pregnancy: Preterm birth from a biobehavioral perspective. *Journal of Midwifery & Women's Health, 54*(1), 8–17. https://doi.org/10.1016/j.jmwh.2008.08.001

Lee, S. K., McMillan, D. D., Ohlsson, A., Boulton, J., Lee, D. S. C., Ting, S., & Liston, R. (2003). The benefit of preterm birth at tertiary care centers is related to gestational age. *American Journal of Obstetrics & Gynecology, 188*(3), 617–622. https://doi.org/10.1067/mob.2003.139

Mackeen, A. D., Seibel-Seamon, J., Muhammad, J., Baxter, J. K., & Berghella, V. (2014). Tocolytics for preterm premature rupture of membranes. *Cochrane Database of Systematic Reviews, 2.* https://doi.org/10.1002/14651858.CD007062.pub3

Marlow, N., Bennett, C., Draper, E. S., Hennessy, E. M., Morgan, A. S., & Costeloe, K. L. (2014). Perinatal outcomes for extremely preterm babies in relation to place of birth in England: The EPICure 2 study. *Archives of Disease in Childhood – Fetal and Neonatal Edition, 99*(3), F181. https://doi.org/10.1136/archdischild-2013-305555

McGoldrick, E., Stewart, F., Parker, R., & Dalziel, S. R. (2020). Antenatal corticosteroids for accelerating fetal lung maturation for women at risk of preterm birth. *Cochrane Database of Systematic Reviews, 12.* https://doi.org/10.1002/14651858.CD004454.pub4

National Institute for Health and Care Excellence. (2015). *Preterm Labour and Birth. NICE Guideline.* Last updated June 2022. Available online: https://www.nice.org.uk/guidance/ng25. Accessed: 20/04/2024

O'Sullivan, C., Heath, P. T., Lamagni, T., Boyle, M., Doherty, L, Reynolds, A., et al. (2015). *Group B Streptococcal Disease in Infants <90 Days of Age..* Available at: www.rcpch.ac.uk/bpsu/gbs. Accessed: 28/04/2024.

Phares, C. R., Lynfield, R., Farley, M. M., Mohle-Boetani, J., Harrison, L. H., Petit, S., Craig, A. S., Schaffner, W., Zansky, S. M., Gershman, K., Stefonek, K. R., Albanese, B. A., Zell, E. R., Schuchat, A., Schrag, S. J., & Active Bacterial Core surveillance/Emerging Infections Program Network (2008). Epidemiology of invasive group B streptococcal disease in the United States, 1999-2005. *JAMA*, *299*(17), 2056–2065. https://doi.org/10.1001/jama.299.17.2056

Porcellato, L., Masson, G., O'Mahony, F., Jenkinson, S., Vanner, T., Cheshire, K., & Perkins, E. (2015). "It's something you have to put up with" —Service users' experiences of *in utero* transfer: A qualitative study. *BJOG: An International Journal of Obstetrics and Gynaecology*, *122*(13), 1825–1832. https://doi.org/10.1111/1471-0528.13235

Rodriguez, A., Wang, Y., Ali Khan, A., Cartwright, R., Gissler, M., & Järvelin, M.-R. (2019). Antenatal corticosteroid therapy (ACT) and size at birth: A population-based analysis using the Finnish Medical Birth Register. *PLOS Medicine*, *16*(2), e1002746. https://doi.org/10.1371/journal.pmed.1002746

Schrag, S. J., Zywicki, S., Farley, M. M., Reingold, A. L., Harrison, L. H., Lefkowitz, L. B., Hadler, J. L., Danila, R., Cieslak, P. R., & Schuchat, A. (2000). Group B streptococcal disease in the era of intrapartum antibiotic prophylaxis. *The New England Journal of Medicine*, *342*(1), 15–20. https://doi.org/10.1056/NEJM200001063420103

Scottish Perinatal Network Transport Group. (2023). *In-Utero Transfers in Scotland Consultant Led Unit to Consultant Led Unit*. https://www.perinatal-network.scot/wp-content/uploads/2023/03/In-Utero-Transfers-in-Scotland-CLU-to-CLU.pdf

Shennan, A., Suff, N., Jacobsson, B., & Birth, the F. W. G. for P. (2021). FIGO good practice recommendations on magnesium sulfate administration for preterm fetal neuroprotection. *International Journal of Gynecology & Obstetrics*, *155*(1), 31–33. https://doi.org/10.1002/ijgo.13856

Shepherd, E., Salam, R. A., Manhas, D., Synnes, A., Middleton, P., Makrides, M., & Crowther, C. A. (2019). Antenatal magnesium sulphate and adverse neonatal outcomes: A systematic review and meta-analysis. *PLOS Medicine*, *16*(12), e1002988. https://doi.org/10.1371/journal.pmed.1002988

Stock, S. J., Thomson, A. J., Papworth, S., & Gynaecologists, the R. C. of O. and. (2022). Antenatal corticosteroids to reduce neonatal morbidity and mortality. *BJOG: An International Journal of Obstetrics & Gynaecology*, *129*(8), e35–e60. https://doi.org/10.1111/1471-0528.17027

Synnes, A., Luu, T. M., Moddemann, D., Church, P., Lee, D., Vincer, M., Ballantyne, M., Majnemer, A., Creighton, D., Yang, J., Sauve, R., Saigal, S., Shah, P., & Lee, S. K. (2017). Determinants of developmental outcomes in a very preterm

Canadian cohort. *Archives of Disease in Childhood – Fetal and Neonatal Edition, 102*(3), F235. https://doi.org/10.1136/archdischild-2016-311228

Thomson, A. J. and RCOG (2019). Care of women presenting with suspected preterm prelabour rupture of membranes from 24+0 weeks of gestation. *BJOG: An International Journal of Obstetrics & Gynaecology, 126*(9), e152–e166. https://doi.org/10.1111/1471-0528.15803

Watson, H., McLaren, J., Carlisle, N., Ratnavel, N., Watts, T., Zaima, A., Tribe, R. M., & Shennan, A. H. (2020). All the right moves: Why *in utero* transfer is both important for the baby and difficult to achieve and new strategies for change [version 1; peer review: 2 approved]. *F1000Research, 9*(979). https://doi.org/10.12688/f1000research.25923.1

World Health Organization. (2022). *WHO Recommendations on Antenatal Corticosteroids for Improving Preterm Birth Outcomes.* https://www.who.int/publications/i/item/9789240057296

Zeitlin, J., Manktelow, B. N., Piedvache, A., Cuttini, M., Boyle, E., van Heijst, A., & *et al.* (2016). Use of evidence based practices to improve survival without severe morbidity for very preterm infants: Results from the EPICE population based cohort. *BMJ, 354.* https://doi.org/10.1136/bmj.i2976

Chapter 7
Care of the woman in threatened preterm labour

Introduction

This chapter describes the care of women with symptoms of threatened preterm labour (TPTL). It outlines the factors midwives should be mindful of when undertaking the initial assessment, clinical investigations, biomarkers tests, transvaginal ultrasound measurement of cervical length, clinical decision support tools and current national guidance.

Initial assessment

On arrival at the assessment unit, women with symptoms of TPTL will be prioritised according to their symptoms, i.e., she will be seen more urgently if she appears to be in established labour or if she reports bleeding. The attending clinicians will undertake an initial assessment which usually involves the below elements:

Assessment of symptoms

Symptoms (such as tightenings and pain) are not reliable indications of which women will go on to deliver early. In Guinn and colleagues' (1997) study of 179 women with symptoms of TPTL, 70%

DOI: 10.4324/9781003380504-7

went on to give birth at term (Guinn *et al.*, 1997). In another study of 763 women with symptoms, more than 95% did not give birth within 14 days of presenting (Peaceman *et al.*, 1997). Symptoms of preterm labour may differ from term labour and may not be as obvious. Clinicians should ask women if are experiencing tightenings, back pain or abdominal pain, but also remember that women may describe these symptoms differently, such as feeling like 'period pain' (Carlisle *et al.*, 2021a, 2021b). Clinicians should therefore avoid simply using medical terminology. It is also important to explore any other symptoms, and whether they think their membranes have ruptured. While it is reassuring to note that most women with symptoms are not in 'true' preterm labour, it is vital to identify and treat, quickly, those who are.

Medical and obstetric history

As in all pregnancy care, an understanding the woman's medical and obstetric history is the foundation upon which the whole assessment is based. The clinician must determine whether the woman has additional risk factors that increase her likelihood of having this baby early (see Chapter 3: Risk factors for spontaneous preterm birth). If she does have risk factors, she may already be under the care of a specialist preterm birth surveillance clinic, and she may already be having treatment (for example, be taking progesterone supplementation or have a cerclage *in situ)*. It is also important to note whether she has presented with similar symptoms before in this pregnancy.

Observations

Midwives should follow their local guidelines on maternal observations, but these are likely to include blood pressure, pulse, temperature, as well as an abdominal palpation, cardiotocograph (CTG) or auscultation of the fetal heart rate, depending on gestation. From a preterm birth perspective, it is important to note any signs or symptoms of infection, particularly if ruptured membranes are suspected, as she and her baby are at increased risk from chorioamnionitis and sepsis.

Speculum examination

A speculum examination may be offered, particularly if the woman reports unusual vaginal discharge. In most UK hospitals, speculum examinations before 37 weeks' gestation are carried out by obstetricians. However, midwives are authorised to carry them out in some units, so it is important to check local policies. It is important to remember that women who have a cerclage *in situ*, cervical (Arabin or vaginal) pessary and/or are using progesterone pessaries can, as a result, experience increased vaginal discharge.

Vaginal swabs can be taken during a speculum examination. These swabs could be for infection screening as well as for predictive biomarker tests, such as fetal fibronectin (this is described more in Chapter 4: Specialist care for the woman at risk). On speculum examination, it may be possible to visualise whether the woman's cervix is opening, and/or if her membranes are visible, or have ruptured. While a closed cervix on speculum is an encouraging sign, it cannot rule out cervical shortening or funnelling. For this, a transvaginal ultrasound scan for cervical length measurement is required.

Predictive biomarker tests

As described in Chapter 4: Specialist care for the woman at risk, biomarker tests can aid decision making when caring for women with symptoms of TPTL, as well as asymptomatic high-risk women. In England, the most commonly used biomarker test is fetal fibronectin (either qualitative, where a result is reported as positive or negative, using a threshold of 50 ng/ml, or quantitative, where the concentration is given between 0 and over 500 ng/ml). Fetal fibronectin testing is used in 76% (71/93) of units for assessing women with symptoms of

TPTL, with most of these (90%; 64/71) using quantitative fetal fibronectin testing (Carlisle *et al.*, 2023).

In women with symptoms of TPTL, the method of taking the fetal fibronectin sample is exactly the same as for asymptomatic women (see Chapter 4: Specialist care for the woman at risk). The sample should be taken before any other manipulation of the cervix (such as a digital vaginal examination or transvaginal cervical length scan) as per the manufacturer's instructions. A fetal fibronectin swab should be taken before these other investigations, but it does not need to be processed immediately. Fetal fibronectin collection swabs are usually supplied free of charge (or at minimal cost) and can be left unprocessed, and at room temperature, for up to 8 hours. The fetal fibronectin test cassettes are relatively expensive, so analysis of the sample can be delayed, and then only run if the woman's full assessment suggests it is necessary. Quantitative fetal fibronectin is validated for use in women with symptoms of TPTL between 22^{+0} and 35^{+6} weeks' gestation.

A smaller percentage of hospitals in England use other biomarker tests, Actim® Partus (16%, 15/93), or PartoSure® (10%, 9/93) (Carlisle *et al.*, 2023). Unlike fetal fibronectin, the evidence base behind their use is currently limited, so they are not recommended by NICE (NICE, 2015). However, due to current fetal fibronectin shortages, Actim® Partus has been recommended by NHS England as an alternative test (NHS England, 2023).

Women do not always feel involved in decision making around whether or not tests are carried out, and may not understand the clinical relevance of fetal fibronectin testing (Carlisle *et al.*, 2021a, 2021b). As in all pregnancy care, time should be taken to ensure that the woman understands the tests offered, and that fully informed consent is obtained before the test is carried out.

Transvaginal ultrasound scan for cervical length measurement

As described in Chapter 4: Specialist care for the woman at risk, transvaginal cervical length scans can also support decision making in care of women with symptoms of TPTL. Cervical length measurement is carried out by 38% (35/93) of hospitals in England as part of the assessment of women with symptoms (Carlisle *et al.*, 2023). This is lower than fetal fibronectin testing because it requires intensive training as well as availability of ultrasound scan equipment. A cervical length scan will determine not just the length of the woman's cervix, but also other characteristics, such as the presence or absence of funnelling or amniotic fluid sludge (see Chapter 4: Specialist care for the woman at risk for more details).

Clinical decision support tool: QUiPP App

The QUiPP App, as described in Chapter 4: Specialist care for the woman at risk can also be used to support decision making when caring for women with symptoms of TPTL. A survey of English maternity units in 2021, showed that just over half of hospitals in England (51%, 47/93) used the QUiPP App when assessing women with symptoms of TPTL (Carlisle et al., 2023). Its use is recommended by the Scottish Perinatal Network (Scottish Perinatal Network Transport Group, 2023), and the London Maternity Clinical Network, in all London hospitals, to identify women requiring *in utero* transfer. In response to the COVID-19 pandemic, and increased need to ensure hospitalisation was offered to those who really needed it, the QUiPP App was also recommended in the care of symptomatic women by NHS England (NHS England, 2020), and a free toolkit was developed to support its implementation (Carlisle *et al.*, 2021a, 2021b). The toolkit is hosted by the British Association of Perinatal Medicine and can be accessed here: www.bapm.org/pages/187-quipp-app-toolkit.

Guidance can vary between maternity units and/or different maternity networks, but most commonly a QUiPP risk of 5% or higher, of preterm delivery within one week of testing is used to determine whether a woman should be admitted, transferred to a hospital with an appropriate level neonatal unit, or discharged home. Using this threshold, the majority of women will be sent home, and these should be reassured that they have a low chance of labouring, but advised to come back if symptoms persist or worsen (Figure 7.1).

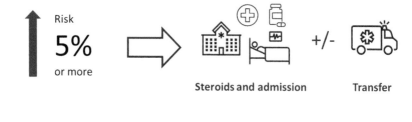

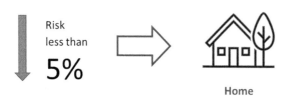

Figure 7.1 Recommended care of women with symptoms of threatened preterm labour, based on QUiPP risk of delivery within seven days

Source: Adapted from BAPM toolkit: www.bapm.org/pages/187-quipp-app-toolkit

Although it is very likely their symptoms will settle, some women can feel confused if they have not received a firm diagnosis or explanation about why they are experiencing these symptoms (Carlisle *et al.*, 2021a, 2021b; Carter *et al.*, 2018).

NICE guidance

Current NICE guidance recommends that all women with suspected preterm labour under 30 weeks should be offered hospital admission and steroids (NICE, 2015). This guidance is summarised in Figure 7.2.

This NICE 'treat-all' policy aims to ensure babies born under 30 weeks' gestation are not inadvertently born outside hospital. However, research has shown that if the QUiPP App was used along with a 5% threshold for management (as described above), 89.4% of unnecessary hospital admissions and associated costs and interventions (such as antenatal corticosteroids) would be safely avoided (Watson *et al.*, 2017).

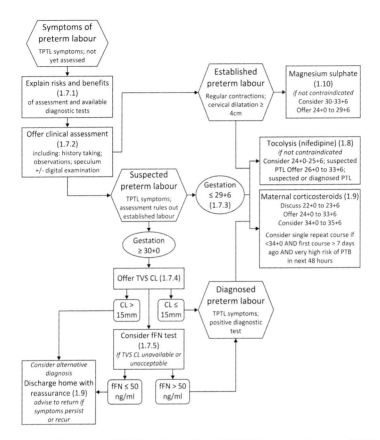

Figure 7.2 Summary of NICE (2015, updated 2022) Preterm Labour and Birth Guideline (NG25) recommendations for women with intact membranes with definitions and guideline section numbers. CL = cervical length; fFN = fetal fibronectin; PTL = preterm labour; TPTL = threatened preterm labour; TVS = transvaginal ultrasound scan

Source: Carter (2019)

Care of women with symptoms before 22 weeks

Care of a woman with symptoms before 22 weeks, when the baby is not expected to survive, if born, will be different, in terms of the interventions to reduce neonatal mortality and morbidity (see Chapter 6: Interventions to improve neonatal outcomes), but the woman's physical and emotional needs are the same. She is still at risk of infection and bleeding, and likely to be extremely anxious at the potential loss of her baby. At these gestations, palliative care will be offered as the baby is not expected to survive (BAPM, 2019). As the earlier the threatened loss occurs, the less common it is, thankfully, but this can mean staff may be inexperienced in caring for women in this scenario (Box 7.1).

Box 7.1 In her own words: woman's experience of mid-trimester loss

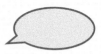

My waters broke early. I rang triage, several times, and each time they told me to wear a sanitary pad. This was not seen as an emergency. I felt unheard.

I went to the GP. He dip-sticked my urine and sent me to the Birth Centre. The midwife lectured me for not ringing first. I was distressed. She examined me, did a swab and told me it was not possible for my waters to break early. She gave me the number for the antenatal yoga teacher and told me to enjoy my pregnancy.

Back at home, I started bleeding clots. No one believed my waters had broken. I went back to the hospital and took the blood clots with me. They sent a student midwife, who could not tell me what the blood clots were. I never felt so scared. The doctor could not tell me either.

I asked for a scan. He tried several times with the scan department, but he could not overrule their decision, I wasn't a priority. He said, you already have a scan booked, go home and wait. I said no.

I fought to be kept in the hospital. It was only when I had a scan, days later, they realised my waters had gone (PPROM), but no one told me this. As a result, infection was missed. I developed sepsis, which led to the loss of my baby.

The midwife did not hand me my baby when she was born. Instead she asked me, but I was too scared of holding her in case she cried. I remember the cries of the other babies, but no cries from my baby. I wished it had been me who died.

I was less than 24 weeks. It was thought my baby couldn't survive. At that point I felt I was nobody's priority.

Ciara, mother to Sinead

There are currently no national clinical guidelines for care of women with threatened mid-trimester loss, but the authors are both members of a guideline development working group, and hope to see these published in the near future.

Summary

In this chapter we have described the care a woman with symptoms of threatened preterm labour may be offered when she arrives at the hospital. This included what the initial assessment may involve, investigations she may be offered, and what current national guidance recommends for women with these symptoms. What midwives should also remember is that women sometimes delay seeking help because they believe they might be worrying unnecessarily (Carlisle *et al.*, 2021a, 2021b). They should be encouraged to always seek advice if they have any concerns, and ensure they know who to contact, and how. This may vary, depending on their gestation (e.g. early pregnancy unit, maternity assessment, labour triage etc.). Women of childbearing age often have busy lives, with work and home responsibilities, which may also contribute their delaying seeking help (Carlisle *et al.*, 2021a, 2021b).

Box 7.2 **Chapter summary and recommendations for practice**

- Threatened preterm labour, and threatened mid-trimester loss, is a worrying and stressful time for mothers and partners.
- Biomarker tests such as fetal fibronectin, cervical length scans and the QUiPP App can help clinicians determine which women require admission and/*or in utero* transfer.
- Women experiencing symptoms before 22 weeks (threatened mid-trimester loss) have the same physical and emotional needs of those having symptoms later.

References

BAPM. (2019). *Perinatal Management of Extreme Preterm Birth before 27 Weeks of Gestation. A BAPM Framework for Practice.* https://www.bapm.org/resources/80-perinatal-management-of-extreme-preterm-birth-before-27-weeks-of-gestation-2019

Carlisle, N., Care, A., Anumba, D. O. C., Dalkin, S., Sandall, J., & Shennan, A. H. (2023). How are hospitals in England caring for women at risk of preterm birth in 2021? The influence of national guidance on preterm birth care in England: A national questionnaire. *BMC Pregnancy and Childbirth, 23*(1), 47. https://doi.org/10.1186/s12884-023-05388-w

Carlisle, N., Watson, H. A., Kuhrt, K., Carter, J., Seed, P. T., Tribe, R. M., Sandall, J., & Shennan, A. H. (2021a). Ten women's decision-making experiences in threatened preterm labour: Qualitative findings from the EQUIPTT trial. *Sexual & Reproductive Healthcare, 100611.* https://doi.org/10.1016/j.srhc.2021.100611

Carlisle, N., Watson, H. A., & Shennan, A. H. (2021b). Development and rapid rollout of the QUiPP App toolkit for women who arrive in threatened preterm labour. *BMJ Open Quality, 10*(2), e001272. https://doi.org/10.1159/000314018

Carter, J. (2019). *Threatened Preterm Labour: A Prospective Cohort Study for the Development of a Clinical Risk Assessment Tool and a Qualitative Exploration of Women's Experiences of Risk Assessment and Management* (Doctoral dissertation, King's College London).

Carter, J., Tribe, R. M., Shennan, A. H., & Sandall, J. (2018). Threatened preterm labour: Women's experiences of risk and care management: A qualitative study. *Midwifery.* https://doi.org/10.1016/j.midw.2018.06.001

Guinn, D. A., Goepfert, A. R., Owen, J., Brumfield, C., & Hauth, J. C. (1997). Management options in women with preterm uterine contractions: A randomized clinical trial. *American Journal of Obstetrics & Gynecology, 177*(4), 814–818. https://doi.org/10.1016/S0002-9378(97)70274-6

NHS England. (2020). *Appendix I: Implications of COVID-19 on Reducing Preterm Births.* https://www.england.nhs.uk/wp-content/uploads/2020/04/C0499-Appx-I-to-SBLCBv2-Reducing-preterm-births.pdf

NHS England. (2023). *Hologic Fetal Fibronectin Cassettes.* Available at: https://www.england.nhs.uk/long-read/hologic-fetal-fibronectin-cassettes/

National Institute for Health and Care Excellence. (2015). *Preterm Labour and Birth. NICE Guideline.* Last updated June 2022. Available online: https://www.nice.org.uk/guidance/ng25 Accessed: 20/04/2024

Peaceman, A. M., Andrews, W. W., Thorp, J. M., Cliver, S. P., Lukes, A., Iams, J. D., Coultrip, L., Eriksen, N., Holbrook, R. H., Elliott, J., Ingardia, C., & Pietrantoni, M. (1997). Fetal fibronectin as a predictor of preterm birth in patients with symptoms: A multicenter trial. *American Journal of Obstetrics and Gynecology*, *177*(1), 13–18. https://doi.org/10.1016/S0002-9378(97)70431-9

Scottish Perinatal Network Transport Group. (2023). *In-Utero Transfers in Scotland Consultant Led Unit to Consultant Led Unit*. https://www.perinatalnetwork.scot/wp-content/uploads/2023/03/In-Utero-Transfers-in-Scotland-CLU-to-CLU.pdf

Watson, H. A., Carter, J., Seed, P. T., Tribe, R. M., & Shennan, A. H. (2017). The QUiPP app: A safe alternative to a treat-all strategy for threatened preterm labor. *Ultrasound in Obstetrics & Gynecology*, *50*(3), 342–346. https://doi.org/10.1002/uog.17499

Chapter 8
Care of the woman in hospital

Introduction

In this chapter, we discuss the care women may receive because their risk of preterm birth is so high they are advised to stay in hospital. Women presenting with symptoms of threatened preterm labour and women attending for specialist preterm care may be admitted if their birth appears imminent, for example, if they are found to have an opening cervix identified on transvaginal ultrasound scan. If there is no appropriate level neonatal unit, or an available cot locally, they may need to be transferred to another hospital (*in utero* transfer). This care will include observations of her own, and her baby's wellbeing, as well as preparation for the birth and what may happen immediately after the birth. Neonatal care of the newborn preterm baby is outside the scope of this book.

As discussed in Chapter 6: Interventions to improve neonatal outcomes, admission to hospital of women who are at high risk of preterm birth is predominantly an intervention to reduce poor outcomes for the baby by ensuring they are born where there is appropriate level of neonatal care. However, hospitalisation may also be appropriate for her own observation and treatment, e.g., if her membranes have ruptured and she is at risk of chorioamnionitis and sepsis. Although the focus of this chapter is on the care of women in hospital with viable pregnancies, many of the principles, particularly those relating to her psychological care, can be applied to those women with symptoms of threatened mid-trimester loss (Box 8.1). This is particularly important if she has been admitted to a gynaecology ward rather than a maternity antenatal ward.

DOI: 10.4324/9781003380504-8

Box 8.1 In her own words: a woman's experience of being in hospital for very high risk of preterm birth

With my first I was in hospital at 25 weeks because my cervix was dilating. I had a rescue suture placed and was to stay in until delivery. I felt really scared. I asked to see someone from the neonatal unit who gave me survival rates, so I knew what to expect.

It was scary and lonely. Your family can only visit during visiting and even then it's hard to talk about the baby not knowing if it's even going to survive. A premature baby can be daunting but not all have health problems so some good examples would provide reassurance. The days are long in hospital and being on a maternity ward, not knowing your baby's fate, can be hard. My son, Olly, was delivered at 27 weeks and five days.

With my second child, Oscar, when I went for my 20-week scan I was told I was dilating. I had another rescue suture but this caused PROM. I tried to keep my son inside, trying to get him to viability. I'd have done anything to give him the best chance, and prevent him being passed to me to die in my arms. But I got sepsis and had to be induced. I felt so guilty. I blamed my body for letting him down, and I'm not sure the medical staff know how soul destroying it is when they are bringing something on that your whole soul wants to stop. He was born at 22 weeks. He survived for five weeks, dying from sepsis caused by his longline. This experience was totally different to the first. I had to beg the doctors and nurses to see why it meant so much to me to try to get my son to viability. I had comments like 'You can have another baby'. All I wanted was empathy. Whatever the gestation it is your baby, whatever the odds are. On this occasion, I found the delivery ward very difficult. The other pregnant women were coming in complaining about getting induced while I just wanted my child to stay inside safe. I asked to be moved off the ward and eventually got my own room. I had suffered with hyperemesis so my pregnancy was horrible. I didn't have a baby shower and now I was in hospital in labour in my early 20s while I watched families coming in full of joy with balloons. I had never had this happy experience – it was upsetting. I found it easier being away from the ward in my own room.

Lauren

Antenatal admission and *in utero* transfer

Once a decision has been made to admit the woman to hospital, the STEAMED mnemonic (Box 8.2) (Carlisle *et al.*, 2020a, 2020b) may be useful for planning her care:

Box 8.2 '**STEAMED**' **care planning mnemonic (from Carlisle *et al.*, 2020a, 2020b)**

1 **S: Steroids**
2 **T: Tocolysis**
3 **E: Early discussion with neonatal team**
4 **A: Antibiotics?** Infection & Group B Streptococcus (GBS) Prophylaxis
5 **M: Magnesium sulphate**
6 **E: Evaluate** – does this woman require *in utero* transfer?
7 **D: Delivery plan**

Consideration should be given to location of the bed allocated to the woman on admission. Ideally, those at risk of preterm birth should not be in the same room as women admitted for induction of labour (Carter *et al.*, 2018).

On admission, observations should be carried out as per local guidelines, whilst the woman is reassured and made to feel as welcome and comfortable as possible. It is important to remember that this is a frightening time for women and their families. If the woman has been transferred from another hospital, she will not just be in an unfamiliar hospital environment but may be geographically far away from family and friends. Women often have conflicting responsibilities (Carter *et al.*, 2018) and may worry about other children at home or work commitments (Carlisle *et al.*, 2021). Women may not have anticipated a hospital admission so may not have additional clothes or toiletries.

The woman and her partner should be provided with information regarding what to expect. Discussions with the neonatal team and visits to the neonatal unit can be arranged so parents can see the machines and environment before their baby is born and quickly taken there after birth.

Maternal breast milk is an important element of the perinatal optimisation care plan (BAPM, 2020a). Midwives should discuss this and other feeding options before the birth, and begin the process of expressing and saving colostrum, if and when the woman is willing.

Clinicians should be mindful of the intense anxiety women and partners may be suffering (Figure 8.1) and offer appropriate mental health support

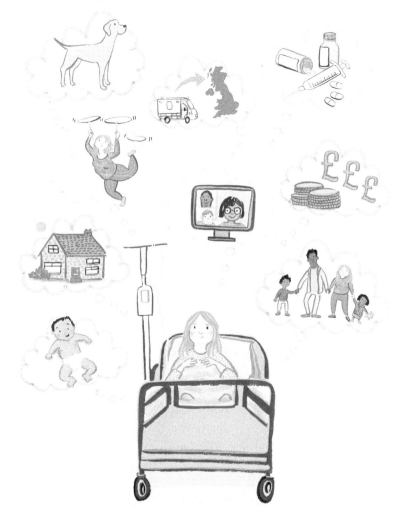

Figure 8.1 Some of the concerns experienced by women in hospital for high risk of preterm birth

Artist: Gemma Baxter

and resources, such as those available through charities like Bliss and Tommy's (https://www.bliss.org.uk/; www.tommys.org). However, not all women, particularly those trying to distract themselves to cope with anxiety, will want to access these. Research has shown that women can struggle with the uncertainty of preterm labour and may not want to consider or discuss potentially poor outcomes (Carter *et al.*, 2018). This can be particularly difficult if they witness other women on the ward, also admitted for preterm birth risk, going on to experience poor outcomes (Carter *et al.*, 2018).

Planning for delivery

As discussed in Chapter 7: Care of the woman in threatened preterm labour, many women admitted for high risk of preterm birth will not go on to deliver early. Symptoms may settle, or they may reach a gestation at which it is safe for them to be discharged home. If they were transferred from another hospital with a lower-level neonatal unit, they may be transferred back if they reach a gestation at which the hospital's neonatal unit can provide care.

Initially, however, a plan and preparations for the birth should be made. This should involve a multidisciplinary team comprising the neonatal, obstetric and midwifery teams as well as the woman and her partner. Discussions will include the mode of birth and whether a caesarean section should be undertaken for fetal indications. This decision will be determined by the gestation of the baby, the estimated fetal weight (if known), fetal and maternal co-morbidities (e.g. cardiac abnormalities, which can reduce the chance of neonatal survival), fetal infection (suspected chorioamnionitis) and parental wishes. The neonatal team will have more significant input in these discussions at earlier preterm gestations, those on the cusp of viability (after 22 weeks' gestation) and those with expected fetal co-morbidities.

The delivery plan should include the following:

- Plan for monitoring (e.g. no monitoring, intermittent auscultation, continuous CTG)
- Mode of delivery
- Indications for caesarean section (and type)
- Neonatal team attendance and plan for resuscitation and stabilisation versus palliative care

The decision whether to offer active management or palliative care for the extremely preterm baby will depend on a variety of factors, based on their chance of survival. When the woman is less than 27 weeks' pregnant, clinicians may find the following infographic decision tool (BAPM, 2019a) helpful (Figure 8.2):

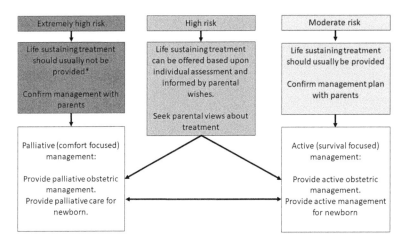

*However, assess for modifiable risk factors and reassess risk if/when circumstances change.

Figure 8.2 Perinatal management of extreme preterm birth before 27 weeks of
          gestation

Source: Adapted from BAPM (2019a)

Intrapartum care of women in preterm labour

If symptoms proceed to established preterm labour, interventions to reduce the risk of neonatal complications (see Chapter 7: Care of the woman in threatened preterm labour) should be commenced, if they have not already. Depending on local guidance, the neonatologists would usually be present at all births from 23^{+0} to 36^{+6} weeks' gestation. The neonatal team may also attend births of babies who are between 22^{+0} and 22^{+6} weeks' gestation, if the decision to provide active management has been made.

Fetal monitoring

There is no national or international guidance on fetal monitoring for women in preterm labour. Recommendations for fetal monitoring when a woman is in preterm labour may therefore differ in local trust guidelines, however in the absence of these, the below recommendations, taken from the Guy's and St Thomas' NHS Foundation Trust guidelines on care of women in threatened preterm labour (Carlisle *et al.*, 2020b) may be helpful.

The guideline recommends that women between 26^{+0} and 36^{+6} weeks' gestation who are contracting regularly and/or in preterm labour should have continuous cardiotocography (CTG) monitoring (not intermittent auscultation). Between 24^{+0} and 25^{+6} weeks' gestation a senior obstetrician should discuss the evidence and aims of fetal heart monitoring with the parents. Before 24^{+0} weeks' gestation, the decision to monitor the fetal heart is usually the consultant obstetrician's decision (after discussion with the neonatal team and parents). In most cases before 24 weeks' gestation this would involve intermittent auscultation by handheld Doppler device ('Sonicaid') or ultrasound scan (Carlisle *et al.*, 2020b). Current NICE guidelines recommend involvement of a senior obstetrician when decisions are made on monitoring the fetal heart rate before 25^{+6} weeks' gestation (NICE, 2015). This is because the interpretation of auscultation findings in term low-risk women cannot be reliably extrapolated to this high-risk group.

Preterm infants are more susceptible to damage caused by intrapartum hypoxia, but characteristics of the CTG trace can vary at different gestations. These variations in CTG characteristics are summarised in Figure 8.3.

In computerised CTG (cCTG) monitoring, ST analyser (or STAN) is not recommended before 36 weeks' gestation as it is unlikely to be reliable (Afors and Chandraharan, 2011).

Fetal scalp electrodes are not recommended before 34^{+0} weeks'. This is following a trend of scalp injuries reported in preterm infants which may be due to preterm infants' more fragile scalp tissue, immature immune system and wider separation of skull bones (de Groot *et al.*, 2013; Gill *et al.*, 1997; Kawakita *et al.*, 2016). However, if external CTG or intermittent auscultation are not possible, the benefits are likely to outweigh potential risks. If the alternatives (i.e. immediate birth, intermittent ultrasound and no monitoring) have been discussed with the woman and are unacceptable to her, then it may be considered (NICE, 2015).

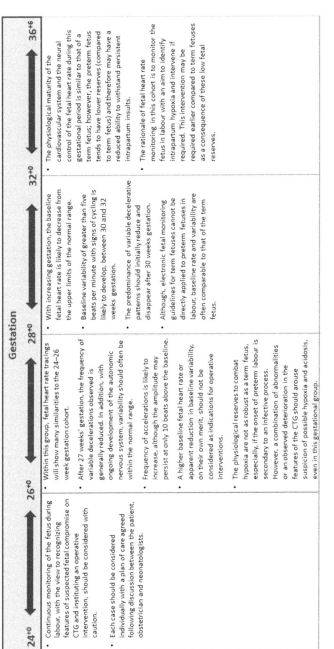

Figure 8.3 Characteristics of fetal heart rate on CTG in the preterm fetus during labour and rationale for monitoring

Source: Adapted from Afors and Chandraharan (2011)

Fetal blood sampling has not been validated in preterm infants (Afors and Chandraharan, 2011). Research has shown that fetal acidosis occurs more frequently in preterm infants delivered before 34 weeks than those delivered between 34 and 36 weeks' gestation (Westgren *et al.*, 1982). Despite this high rate of fetal acidosis, however, the infant outcomes in the short-term were good, and in later repeat blood sampling the pH values had normalised (Westgren *et al.*, 1982). It is possible that the high fetal acidosis in preterm infants is an alternative intrapartum compensatory mechanism (Afors and Chandraharan, 2011). However, fetal blood sampling results from infants born between 34 and 36 weeks' gestation, appear to be similar to results from term infants. Therefore, NICE (2015) does not recommend fetal blood sampling in woman less than 34^{+0} weeks pregnant.

Amniotomy

Amniotomy should be avoided in women in preterm labour, as it can accelerate premature delivery and lead to compound and abnormal presentations (Carlisle *et al.*, 2020b). Preterm infants delivered in the membranes are also less likely to sustain neonatal bruising. However, if the fetal heart rate is abnormal and delivery is recommended, amniotomy may be appropriate.

Delivery care of women in preterm labour

Optimal cord management

The Resuscitation Council UK, NICE *and* BAPM recommend clinicians wait at least 60 seconds before clamping the cord of preterm babies ('optimal cord management') unless there are specific maternal or fetal conditions or requirements which mean earlier clamping is preferable (Fawke *et al.*, 2021; NICE, 2015; BAPM 2020b). This is because optimal cord management reduces death in preterm babies by 28% (Fogarty *et al.*, 2018). The number of babies needing to receive optimal cord management to prevent one death is around 30–50; however, this could be as low as 20 in the most premature babies (BAPM, 2020b;

Fogarty *et al.*, 2018; Rabe *et al.*, 2019). The BAPM Optimal Cord Management Toolkit has resources which can aid implementation (BAPM, 2020b).

Normothermia

Infant hypothermia is defined as a core body temperature of <36.5°C, or a skin temperature of <36.0°C (World Health Organization, 1997). Preterm babies are at increased risk of hypothermia and its related unfavourable effects (such as hypoglycaemia, hypoxia and metabolic acidosis, respiratory distress and chronic lung disease, necrotising enterocolitis, intraventricular haemorrhage, late-onset sepsis and death (McCall *et al.*, 2018).

Heat can be lost through numerous different routes. There are a broad range of approaches to reduce heat loss and promote normothermia. The BAPM 'Improving Normothermia in Very Preterm Infants' toolkit contains resources to support maternity units to improve care (BAPM, 2019b). For example, to prevent evaporation from warm wet skin at birth, clinicians are advised to deliver preterm infants under 32 weeks' gestation into an occlusive plastic wrap/bag, and ensure the baby wears a woollen or plastic hat (Fawke *et al.*, 2021). Infants over 32 weeks' gestation should be dried and covered with a warm towel (Fawke *et al.*, 2021). To prevent evaporation from the respiratory tract, clinicians can resuscitate with warm, humidified gases (BAPM, 2019b). To prevent heat loss through convection (heat loss due to cooler circulating air), room temperature should be increased to 23–26°C for all deliveries under 32 weeks' gestation, and windows and doors closed (BAPM 2019b). To prevent heat loss through conduction (heat loss due to direct contact with cooler surfaces) a transwarmer or exothermic mattress could be used. Finally, to prevent heat loss due to radiation (which is the non-direct transfer of heat to cooler mediums) it is recommended that a radiant heat source is utilised (BAPM, 2019b).

Maternal breast milk

Maternal breast milk (MBM) for preterm infants has numerous benefits which are outlined in Figure 8.4.

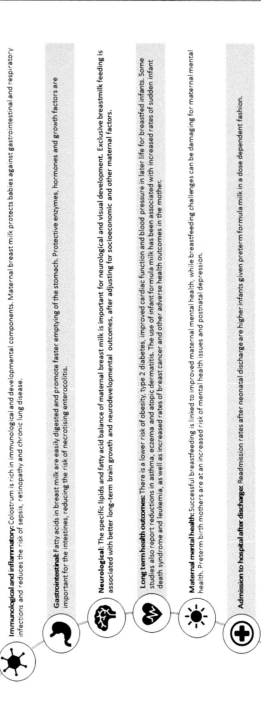

Figure 8.4 The impact of maternal breast milk for preterm babies

Source: Adapted from BAPM (2020a)

If a woman is keen to breastfeed she should be supported and encouraged to do so. The BAPM 'Optimising Early Maternal Breast Milk for Preterm: A Quality Improvement Toolkit' is another resource to support maternity units improve breastfeeding rates (BAPM, 2020a). The resource suggests five perinatal elements to support early maternal breast milk (MBM) for preterm infants (Box 8.2). These can be discussed with the women at high risk of preterm birth during her stay on the antenatal ward.

Box 8.2 **Perinatal elements to support early maternal breast milk for preterm infants (from BAPM, 2020a)**

1 Parents as equal partners in their baby's care: Parents are empowered to take part in all elements of their baby's care, facilitating strong close and loving attachments.

2 Antenatal education: Educating families about the value of MBM in prematurity, importance and process of early expressing.

3 Initiation of expressing soon after birth (aim within 2 hours): With easy access to support, training and equipment.

4 Early colostrum (ideally within 6 hours of birth and always within 24 hours): MBM to be the first enteral feed given to baby.

5 Early and regular parental physical contact with their baby: Delivery room contact, skin-to-skin early and often.

Prehospital management of preterm infants

It is most likely that midwives reading this book will be caring for women in preterm labour in a hospital environment. However, if a midwife finds herself looking after a woman with an imminent preterm birth outside hospital the recommendations from the BAPM 'Pre-hospital management of the baby born at extreme preterm gestation framework' (BAPM, 2022) will be useful. These recommendations are summarised in Box 8.3.

Box 8.3 Recommendations for the care of women during extreme preterm birth outside hospital (adapted from BAPM, 2022)

Preterm birth under 22 weeks' gestation

- If gestation is known to be less than 22 completed weeks (up to and including 21 weeks and 6 days), even if there are signs of life at delivery then resuscitation should not be attempted.
- The focus should be on care for the mother, and comfort care (palliative care) for the baby.
- Parents should be made aware that their baby may show signs of life after birth. The parents should be given time together with their baby, and their wishes on how they want to be involved in their baby's care should be respected. This could include cuddling the baby, taking photographs and other memory making.
- If a midwife is present and the mother is deemed to be stable, then the family may wish to remain at home. If not, then both mother and baby should be transported together to the maternity unit.

Preterm birth after 22 weeks' gestation

- From 22^{+0} weeks' gestation, or if gestation is not known, simple interventions focussed on maintaining body temperature and supporting the airway and breathing should be undertaken. This includes minimising draughts and putting a heater on, and ideally delivering the baby into a polythene bag without drying them first. If there is no bag available, then the baby should be gently dried and wrapped in a warm towel.
- A hat should be placed on the baby (if this not available then an adult large-sized sock could be used instead).
- At least 60 seconds should have passed before the cord is clamped.

- Resuscitation following Newborn Life Support (NLS) principles should be followed. If there is a very slow (<60 bpm) or undetectable heart rate in spite of appropriate airway and breathing support, the BAPM framework outlines that chest compressions will most likely not be helpful and are therefore not recommended below 24^{+0} weeks' gestation. It is most likely that the baby will not survive.
- For babies over 24 weeks' gestation, or where gestation is not known NLS guidance should be followed. If the heart rate stays very slow after 30 seconds of appropriate ventilation, then proceed to chest compressions in a ratio of 3:1 with ventilation, 30 cycles per minute.
- The baby should be reassessed every 2–3 minutes while aiming to maintain temperature. An ambulance and paramedic support should hopefully be present at delivery, or if not, they will hopefully arrive soon after.
- Once initial resuscitation has taken place and if the decision is to transfer, then the mother and baby can be moved to the ambulance.

Summary

In this chapter, the care of women admitted to hospital because they are at very high risk of imminent preterm birth has been discussed. This has included assessment of their and their baby's wellbeing, as well as preparation for the birth and some elements of intrapartum care. Extreme preterm birth outside hospital has also been considered. Neonatal care of the newborn preterm baby has not been discussed in detail as this is beyond the scope of this book. Postnatal care of the woman who has experienced preterm birth or mid-trimester loss is also not covered in this book. That said it should, of course, be provided with sensitivity, and the midwife should be mindful of the challenges the woman may have faced, both before, during and after the birth.

Box 8.4 Chapter summary and recommendations
for practice

- A multidisciplinary plan for delivery should be made with the parents in case preterm labour continues.
- Women above 26 weeks' gestation are recommended to have CTG monitoring in labour.
- Fetal scalp electrodes and fetal blood sampling is not recommended under 34 weeks' gestation.
- All preterm babies should have delayed cord clamping of at least 60 seconds.
- Preterm infants born less than 32 weeks' gestation should be delivered into a plastic bag/polyethylene wrapping.
- Maternal breast milk has many benefits for preterm infants and women who wish to breastfeed their preterm baby should be supported and encouraged to do so.
- If attending a birth outside of the hospital environment, then resuscitation should not be attempted on a baby born less than 22 weeks' gestation.

References

Afors, K., & Chandraharan, E. (2011). Use of continuous electronic fetal monitoring in a preterm fetus: Clinical dilemmas and recommendations for practice. *Journal of Pregnancy, 2011*, 848794. https://doi.org/10.1155/2011/848794

BAPM. (2019a). *Perinatal Management of Extreme Preterm Birth before 27 Weeks of Gestation. A BAPM Framework for Practice.* https://www.bapm.org/resources/80-perinatal-management-of-extreme-preterm-birth-before-27-weeks-of-gestation-2019

BAPM. (2019b). *Improving Normothermia in Very Preterm Infants, A Quality Improvement Toolkit.* Available at: https://hubble-live-assets.s3.amazonaws.com/bapm/redactor2_assets/files/831/OCM_Toolkit_Full_For_Launch.pdf. Accessed: 24/02/2024.

BAPM. (2020a). *Optimising Early Maternal Breast Milk for Preterm Infants A Quality Improvement Toolkit.* Available at: https://hubble-live-assets.s3.amazonaws.com/bapm/redactor2_assets/files/755/BAPM_Preterm_MBM_Toolkit_Final_for_publication.pdf. Accessed: 24/02/2024.

BAPM. (2020b). *Optimal Cord Management in Preterm Babies, A Quality Improvement Toolkit*. Available at: https://hubble-live-assets.s3.amazonaws. com/bapm/redactor2_assets/files/831/OCM_Toolkit_Full_For_Launch.pdf. Accessed: 23/02/2024.

BAPM. (2022). *Pre-Hospital Management of the Baby Born at Extreme Preterm Gestation A Framework for Practice*. Available at: https://hubble-live-assets. s3.eu-west-1.amazonaws.com/bapm/file_asset/file/1120/Prehospital_man-agement_V1.1_May_2022.pdf. Accessed: 25/02/2024.

Carlisle, N., Watson, H. A., & Shennan, A. H. (2020a). *The QUiPP App Toolkit for Women Who Arrive in Threatened Preterm Labour*. Available at: https://www. bapm.org/pages/187-quipp-app-toolkit. Accessed: 23/02/2024.

Carlisle, N., Chandiramani, M., Suff, N., Story, L., Glazewska-Hallin, A., & Shennan, A. 2020b. *Threatened Preterm Labour: Guideline for Management*. Guy's and St Thomas' NHS Foundation Trust.

Carlisle, N., Watson, H. A., Kuhrt, K., Carter, J., Seed, P. T., Tribe, R. M., Sandall, J., & Shennan, AH. (2021). Ten women's decision-making experiences in threatened preterm labour: Qualitative findings from the EQUIPTT trial. *Sexual & Reproductive Healthcare*, *29*, 100611. https://www.sciencedirect. com/science/article/pii/S1877575621000185?via%3Dihub

Carter, J., Tribe, R. M., Shennan, A. H., & Sandall, J. (2018). Threatened preterm labour: Women's experiences of risk and care management: A qualitative study. *Midwifery*. https://doi.org/10.1016/j.midw.2018.06.001

de Groot, P. F., Mol, B. W. J., & Onland, W. (2013). Complications of fetal scalp electrode placement: A case report, literature review and summary of case reports. *Expert Review of Obstetrics & Gynecology*, *8*(2), 113–120. https:// doi.org/10.1159/000314018

Fogarty, M., Osborn, D. A., & Askie, L., *et al*. Delayed vs early umbilical cord clamping for preterm infants: A systematic review and meta-analysis. *American Journal of Obstetrics & Gynecology* 2018;*218*(1):1–18. https://doi. org/10.1016/j.ajog.2017.10.231

Fawke, J., Wyllie, J., Madar, J., Ainsworth, S., Tinnion, R., Chittick, R., Wenlock, N., Cusack, J., Monnelly, V., Lockey, A., & Hampshire, S. (2021). *Newborn Resuscitation and Support of Transition of Infants at Birth Guidelines*. https://www.resus.org.uk/library/2021-resuscitation-guidelines/newborn-resuscitation-and-support-transition-infants-birth

Gill, P., Sobeck, J., Jarjoura, D., Hiller, S., & Benedetti, T. (1997). Mortality from early neonatal group B streptococcal sepsis: Influence of obstetric factors. *Journal of Maternal-Fetal Medicine*, *6*(1), 35–39. https://doi.org/10.1159/000314018

Kawakita, T., Reddy, U. M., Landy, H. J., Iqbal, S. N., Huang, C. C., & Grantz, K. L. (2016 Oct). Neonatal complications associated with use of fetal scalp electrode: A retrospective study. *BJOG*, *123*(11):1797–803. https://doi.org/10.1111/1471-0528.13817. Epub 2015 Dec 8. PMID: 26643181; PMCID: PMC4899296.

McCall, E. M., Alderdice, F., & Vohara, S., *et al.* (2018). Interventions to prevent hypothermia at birth in preterm and/or low birthweight infants. *Cochrane Database of Systematic Reviews*, (2), Art No.: CD004210. https://doi.org/10.1002/14651858.CD004210.pub5

National Institute for Health and Care Excellence. (2015). *Preterm Labour and Birth. NICE Guideline*. Last updated June 2022. Available online: https://www.nice.org.uk/guidance/ng25. Accessed: 20/04/2024.

Rabe, H., Gyte, G. M., & Díaz-Rossello, J. L., *et al.* (2019). Effect of timing of umbilical cord clamping and other strategies to influence placental transfusion at preterm birth on maternal and infant outcomes. *Cochrane Database of Systematic Reviews*;9(9), Cd003248. https://doi.org/10.1002/14651858.CD003248.pub4

Westgren, M., Holmquist, P., Svenningsen, N. W., & Ingemarsson, I. 1982. Intrapartum fetal monitoring in preterm deliveries: Prospective study. *Obstetrics & Gynecology*, *60*(1), 99–106. https://doi.org/10.1159/000314018

World Health Organization. 1997. *Maternal and Newborn Health/Safe Motherhood. Thermal Protection of the Newborn: A Practical Guide*. WHO, Geneva.

Chapter 9

What the future may hold for preterm birth care

Introduction

In the future, people may look back and think that our efforts to explain, let alone prevent, preterm birth were very naïve. Progress in medicine moves forward, sometimes very quickly. As discussed in previous chapters, the *Saving Babies Lives Care Bundle* and other national guidelines should reduce variation in care and lead to more women being identified early and offered appropriate care to reduce in preterm birth and its consequences. Although this advancement in care is welcome, there is a lot more work to be done.

Potential new ways to identify women at risk

Current methods for identifying women at risk largely depend on the presence or absence of risk factors; the most significant of these are previous experience of mid-trimester pregnancy loss and/or spontaneous preterm birth. However, many preterm babies are born to women with no known risk factors; half of these are having their first baby (Iams et al., 2001), so the quest for better predictive tools is urgently needed. A potential change in practice could be introducing cervical length screening to all women in their first pregnancy. However, currently the evidence base to support this strategy is inadequate (Rosenbloom *et al.*, 2020).

DOI: 10.4324/9781003380504-9

Potential novel biomarkers

Fetal fibronectin testing is helpful in supporting management decisions, but it is currently only validated for use from 18 weeks' gestation in high risk, asymptomatic women and from 22 to 23 weeks' in those with symptoms. Research is underway seeking and evaluating potential new biomarkers that may be used earlier in pregnancy. This includes work investigating the vaginal microbiome (Correia *et al.*, 2023; Flaviani *et al.*, 2021; Leow *et al.*, 2020), infection markers (Vakili *et al.*, 2021) and genetics (Wadon *et al.*, 2020). In addition to cervical length, other cervical characteristics may prove to be useful for predicting those most at risk. These include cervical stiffness (Breuking *et al.*, 2023) and uterocervical angle (Hessami *et al.*, 2021). The significance of the uterocervical angle has been suggested as a potential explanation as to why the cervical (Arabin or vaginal) pessary appears to work for some women (Arabin and Alfirevic, 2013). Other potentially useful factors include new ultrasonic markers, including the presence of amniotic fluid sludge (Sapantzoglou *et al.*, 2023) and previous caesarean section scar characteristics (Banerjee *et al.*, 2022).

Advances in the understanding of genetics could also provide novel biomarkers for prediction of preterm birth. Research suggests that cell-free fetal DNA may, later in pregnancy, be an indication that labour is imminent (Dugoff *et al.*, 2016) allowing appropriate intervention, such as administration of steroids and admission to hospital. While DNA replicates and stores genetic information, RNA carries out instructions coded in the DNA. Cell-free RNA has also been shown to be a promising candidate as a prediction marker (Camunas-Soler *et al.*, 2022).

Improvements in technology

If history has anything to tell us, ultrasound and MRI techniques will probably become more sophisticated, machines will probably become smaller and the service, as a whole, relatively less expensive. This could allow us to more efficiently explore, for example, cervical consistency, the position and characteristics of a previous in-labour caesarean section scar and other damage. This could help us to identify women at risk of mid-trimester loss and spontaneous preterm birth earlier, who could then be offered more effective treatments, before they have lost even one baby. Vaginally placed cerclages do not appear to be as effective in these women (Hickland *et al.*, 2020) so transabdominal cerclage may be a more effective treatment.

Another potentially useful biomarker, in the form of tiny microRNA molecules detectable in maternal blood samples, may be able to identify women at risk of preterm birth early in the second trimester (Cook *et al.*, 2019). MicroRNAs help cells to control the type and quantity of the proteins they make (gene expression), which in turn regulate all physiological functions, including regulation of the immune response. Identification of these molecules is very complex and expensive, but work has begun on developing a bedside lateral flow test analyser (Petrou *et al.*, 2022).

Use of healthcare records, big data and computer-assisted intelligence (AI)

As health records have become increasingly electronic, there is the potential for routine records to be used for research purposes. One of the aims of NHS Digital (now incorporated into NHS England) is to allow exploration of this potentially valuable data. However, digital maturity (the readiness of an organisation to integrate digital technologies) across the NHS remains varied and is often sub-optimal (Cresswell *et al.*, 2021; Sheikh et al., 2021). Health professionals in other hospitals, GPs, and sometimes even community midwives working in the same NHS Trust, are unable to access the central maternity records for the women in their care. Hopefully this situation will improve in the future, and that different IT systems are at least harmonised, not just to improve care but also to make it easier for the data to be used in research. This would accelerate the identification of novel risk factors, and combinations of risk factors, that could lead to better targeting of surveillance and interventions for women at risk of preterm birth. Work is already underway exploring how machine learning could utilise 'big data' for predicting preterm birth (Surendiran *et al.*, 2022; Zhang *et al.*, 2022) and this is likely to continue as the quality of data improves. Using healthcare data in this way is likely to lead to more personalisation in all areas of healthcare.

Collaborative working

A sense of collaboration and keenness to share data, amongst researchers in the field through clinical networks, such as the UK Preterm Clinical Network (www.medscinet.net/ukpcn) and the Tommy's National Centre for Preterm Birth Research [https://www.tommys.org/our-research/our-research-centres/tommys-national-centre-preterm-birth-research], provide hope for the future. Clinical databases, such as the Preterm Clinical Network (PCN) Database, already exist (Carter et al., 2018) (see also Chapter 4: Specialist care for the woman at risk). This database can be used to collect data that is more detailed, and relevant to preterm birth, than most electronic maternity records. Data collected through this type of specific clinical database can be linked to routinely collected records, through projects such as the Early Life Cross Linkage in Research (eLIXIR) Partnership (Carson et al., 2020). These records could then be used for research into, for example, combinations of risk factors, long-term outcomes following preterm birth and the safety of interventions designed to prevent it.

More accurately predicting who is most at risk, and likely to benefit from intervention, is crucial to reducing rates of preterm birth. The multifaceted nature of the problem will require a multifaceted approach to overcome it, where researchers share knowledge and work together (Lamont et al., 2020; Vidal et al., 2022).

Potential new interventions to prevent preterm birth

Currently, apart from cerclage and progesterone in women at high risk (Alfirevic et al., 2017; Stewart et al., 2021), few interventions have been shown to prevent preterm birth (Medley et al., 2018). Those that do appear to work, for some, are by no means universally successful, and the search for novel interventions continues. Although it takes many years to develop and thoroughly evaluate new therapies, there are some potential candidates currently under investigation.

Pravastatin

As it appears that labour is triggered by an inflammatory response, it makes sense to consider treatments that might address this. One potential intervention is pravastatin, which is one of a group of medicines called statins. Statins are used to prevent stroke and heart disease as they have a protective effect on blood vessels and reduce inflammation. Unlike other statins, pravastatin does not pass easily across the placenta to the fetus. In previous trials evaluating its use to prevent or treat other problems in pregnancy (i.e. preeclampsia and anti-phospholipid syndrome), there were no safety concerns and it appeared to reduce the number of babies born preterm (Costantine *et al.*, 2016; Lefkou *et al.*, 2016). Pravastatin is currently being evaluated as a preterm prevention intervention in a randomised controlled trial, called PIONEER (https://bristol-trials-centre.bristol.ac.uk/details-of-studies/pioneer/).

Encouraging a healthy vaginal microbiome

As certain 'communities' of microorganisms which make up the vaginal microbiome appear to be protective against preterm birth, it is possible that interventions could be developed to counter overgrowth of pathogenic bacteria and encourage growth of protective communities (Vieira-Baptista *et al.*, 2022). These interventions may include probiotics (live bacteria and yeasts that are intended promote health), or vaginal microbiome transplantation, where the protective *Lactobacillus*-dominated species are introduced from healthy donor vaginal fluid (Lev-Sagie *et al.*, 2019). To date, however, although commercially available and popular, there is currently insufficient evidence to suggest probiotics are effective in preventing preterm birth (Jarde *et al.*, 2018).

Omega-3

Omega-3 fatty acids, commonly found in fish and fish oils, have for some time been proposed as an intervention to prevent preterm birth, but they have not yet become widely used. However, a recent clinical practice guideline has been published following a review of the evidence and expert consensus (Cetin *et al.*, 2023). The consortium of international doctors and scientists recommend all women of child-bearing age should take at least 250 mg daily through diet or supplements and increase this by an additional 100–200 mg per day in pregnancy.

Research

Clinical research in the NHS

The National Institute for Health Research (NIHR) was established in 2006. This is a UK Government-funded body that supports NHS health and social care research in England through funding research projects and people, through fellowships. NIHR Research Delivery Network (RDN) also supports NHS research by co-ordinating and supporting the delivery of research in NHS and care organisations. This includes funding research midwives who may support several studies by identifying and recruiting eligible participants. In the devolved nations, Scotland, Wales and Northern Ireland, arrangements are different, and healthcare research is the responsibility of the Scottish Government's Chief Scientist Office, Health and Care Research Wales and Health and Social Care Research and Development in Northern Ireland.

Research governance is managed locally through hospital R&D (Research and Development) Departments, who guide researchers through the process of approvals, which include HRA (Health Research Authority) and REC (Research Ethics Committee) approvals. Research midwives often work closely with clinical colleagues and are usually very keen to share their knowledge and expertise. If you are interested in research, just to learn more about what is going on in your hospital, or to find how to get more involved, then we would recommend that you contact these research midwives. Reproductive Health and Childbirth is one of the most active areas of research supported by the NIHR. This research includes a variety of research, both qualitative and quantitative, using a range of methodologies. Health service users are often keen to participate in research (Box 9.1), and there is evidence to suggest that patients receiving care in research-active hospitals have better outcomes, even if they are not taking part in research themselves (Ozdemir *et al.*, 2015).

Box 9.1 In her own words: woman's experience of taking part in preterm birth research

'Our last experiences at our previous hospital had been pretty dire. And here at this clinic we had access to the latest tests and also the latest research trials we were put in, but mainly as well by the team that we were surrounded by, the midwives, the doctors, the sonographers, that ladies that made the cups of tea.

Everyone really genuinely cared about our experience there and about us having a successful outcome. We lost our first two girls in April 2010 and in April 2011, Emilia and Grace, and I can't explain how it felt to a) be in a different hospital and b) have this completely different experience to what we'd had before.

It especially gave me, a real sense of purpose, being part of the research trials that were run from the clinic, and it felt like the awful experiences we'd been though was being put to good use. With the knowledge that we could prevent future preterm births happening for other people, as well as ourselves.

But the main thing about being part of this clinic – and you really did feel part of it – was that you had someone fighting your corner for you and they all really, genuinely cared, about every family going in...

Preterm clinics are an absolutely vital part of our NHS. I didn't have access to one locally, and it was more by chance that I could refer [myself] to this one... I've got two bouncing boys as a result of it. Losing my two girls wasn't in vain. It was awful, and horrendous, but you know, it's my four year old's birthday today, and I wouldn't have had him without it.'

Sarah

Implementation Science

Advances in healthcare can only come about through the creation and testing of new knowledge through research and service evaluation. This includes not just evaluation of interventions and whether they work but research into how to get these new interventions successfully into practice. This scientific study of the methods and strategies needed to successful implement evidence-based practice is known as Implementation Science (Bauer and Kirchner, 2020). This is important because there are many factors and contexts that influence whether implementation of a new practice or intervention is successful or not, even if the intervention itself is known to be effective. Identifying and addressing those factors can make a big difference to the success or failure of wider scale up.

Collecting and publishing service indicators, such as rates of caesarean sections, can also encourage compliance with guidelines and implementation of evidence-based care, e.g. through the NHS England Maternity Services Dataset and the National Maternity Dashboard. This allows 'bench-marking', where maternity service providers, and the public, can review individual NHS Trusts and compare their service with others.

Summary

In this chapter, we have discussed some potential future advancements for the care of women at risk of preterm birth. Any improvements in care will depend on robust evidence to support changes in practice. Midwives and the women in their care can get involved in clinical research, and we would encourage all to do so. Without involvement of the women and families who will be impacted by the research, and clinicians who will be implementing the new practices, innovations are less likely to succeed.

Box 9.2 **Chapter summary and recommendations for practice**

- New ways for more accurately predicting and preventing preterm birth are under development.
- Advances in technology and data (AI) could lead to better outcomes for women and their babies.
- Collaborative research is more likely to find answers to the complex and multifaceted problem of preterm birth prediction and prevention.
- Find out what research projects are ongoing in your hospital and get involved by referring eligible women to local research midwives.
- Share your ideas for improvements in practice with local researchers and associated university academics.

References

Alfirevic, Z., Stampalija, T., & Medley, N., 2017. Cervical stitch (cerclage) for preventing preterm birth in singleton pregnancy. *Cochrane Database of Systematic Reviews*, (6).

Arabin, B., & Alfirevic, Z. 2013. Cervical pessaries for prevention of spontaneous preterm birth: Past, present and future. *Ultrasound in Obstetrics & Gynecology*, *42*(4), 390–399. https://doi.org/10.1159/000314018

Banerjee, A., Al-Dabbach, Z., Bredaki, F. E., Casagrandi, D., Tetteh, A., Greenwold, N., Ivan, M., Jurkovic, D., David, A. L., & Napolitano, R. 2022. Reproducibility of assessment of full-dilatation Cesarean section scar in women undergoing second-trimester screening for preterm birth. *Ultrasound in Obstetrics & Gynecology*, *60*(3), 396–403. https://doi.org/10.1159/000314018

Bauer, M. S., & Kirchner, J. 2020. Implementation science: What is it and why should I care? *Psychiatry Research*, *283*, 112376.

Breuking, S., Oudijk, M. A., van Eekelen, R., de Boer, M. A., Pajkrt, E., & Hermans, F. 2023. Assessment of cervical softening and the prediction of preterm birth (STIPP): Protocol for a prospective cohort study. *BMJ Open*, *13*(11), e071597. https://doi.org/10.1159/000314018

Camunas-Soler, J., Gee, E. P., Reddy, M., Dai Mi, J., Thao, M., Brundage, T., Siddiqui, F., Hezelgrave, N. L., Shennan, A. H., Namsaraev, E., & Haverty, C. 2022. Predictive RNA profiles for early and very early spontaneous preterm birth. *American Journal of Obstetrics and Gynecology*, *227*(1), 72–e1. https://doi.org/10.1159/000314018

Carson, L. E., Azmi, B., Jewell, A., Taylor, C. L., Flynn, A., Gill, C., Broadbent, M., Howard, L., Stewart, R., & Poston, L. 2020. Cohort profile: The eLIXIR partnership—A maternity–child data linkage for life course research in South London, UK. *BMJ Open*, *10*(10), e039583. https://doi.org/10.1159/000314018

Carter, J., Tribe, R. M., Sandall, J., & Shennan, A. H. 2018. The preterm clinical network (PCN) database: A web-based systematic method of collecting data on the care of women at risk of preterm birth. *BMC Pregnancy and Childbirth*, *18*, 1–9.

Cetin, I., Carlson, S. E., Burden, C., da Fonseca, E. B., di Renzo, G. C., Hadjipanayis, A., Harris, W. S., Kumar, K. R., Olsen, S. F., Mader, M. S., & McAuliffe, F. M., 2023. Omega-3 fatty acid supply in pregnancy for risk reduction of preterm and early preterm birth. *American Journal of Obstetrics & Gynecology MFM*, *6*(2), 101251.

Cook, J., Bennett, P. R., Kim, S. H., Teoh, T. G., Sykes, L., Kindinger, L. M., Garrett, A., Binkhamis, R., MacIntyre, D. A., & Terzidou, V. 2019. First trimester circulating microRNA biomarkers predictive of subsequent preterm delivery and cervical shortening. *Scientific Reports*, *9*(1), 5861. https://doi.org/10.1159/000314018

Correia, G. D., Marchesi, J. R., & MacIntyre, D. A. 2023. Moving beyond DNA: Towards functional analysis of the vaginal microbiome by non-sequencing-based methods. *Current Opinion in Microbiology*, *73*, 102292.

Costantine, M. M., Cleary, K., & Hebert, M. F., *et al*. 2016. Safety and pharmacokinetics of pravastatin used for the prevention of preeclampsia in high-risk pregnant women: A pilot randomized controlled trial. *American Journal of Obstetrics and Gynecology*, *214*, 720.e721–720.e717.

Cresswell, K., Williams, R., & Sheikh, A. 2021. Bridging the growing digital divide between NHS England's hospitals. *Journal of the Royal Society of Medicine*, *114*(3), 111–112. https://doi.org/10.1159/000314018

Dugoff, L., Barberio, A., Whittaker, P. G., Schwartz, N., Sehdev, H., & Bastek, J. A. 2016. Cell-free DNA fetal fraction and preterm birth. *American Journal of Obstetrics and Gynecology*, *215*(2), 231–e1. https://doi.org/10.1159/000314018

Flaviani, F., Hezelgrave, N. L., Kanno, T., Prosdocimi, E. M., Chin-Smith, E., Ridout, A. E., von Maydell, D. K., Mistry, V., Wade, W. G., Shennan, A. H., & Dimitrakopoulou, K., 2021. Cervicovaginal microbiota and metabolome predict preterm birth risk in an ethnically diverse cohort. *JCI Insight*, *6*(16).

Hessami, K., Kasraeian, M., Sepúlveda-Martínez, Á, Parra-Cordero, M. C., Vafaei, H., Asadi, N., & Benito Vielba, M. 2021. The novel ultrasonographic marker of uterocervical angle for prediction of spontaneous preterm birth in singleton and twin pregnancies: A systematic review and meta-analysis. *Fetal Diagnosis and Therapy*, *48*(2), 81–87. https://doi.org/10.1159/000314018

Hickland, M. M., Story, L., Glazewska-Hallin, A., Suff, N., Cauldwell, M., Watson, H. A., Carter, J., Duhig, K. E., & Shennan, A. H. 2020. Efficacy of transvaginal cervical cerclage in women at risk of preterm birth following previous emergency cesarean section. *Acta Obstetricia et Gynecologica Scandinavica*, *99*(11), 1486–1491. https://doi.org/10.1159/000314018

Iams, J. D., Goldenberg, R. L., Mercer, B. M., Moawad, A. H., Meis, P. J., & Das, A. F., *et al*. 2001. The preterm prediction study: Can low-risk women destined for spontaneous preterm birth be identified? *American Journal of Obstetrics and Gynecology*, *184*(4), 652–655.

Jarde, A., Lewis-Mikhael, A. M., Moayyedi, P., Stearns, J. C., Collins, S. M., Beyene, J., & McDonald, S. D. 2018. Pregnancy outcomes in women taking probiotics or prebiotics: A systematic review and meta-analysis. *BMC Pregnancy and Childbirth*, *18*(1), 1–14. https://doi.org/10.1159/000314018

Lamont, R. F., Richardson, L. S., Boniface, J. J., Cobo, T., Exner, M. M., Christensen, I. B., Forslund, S. K., Gaba, A., Helmer, H., Jørgensen, J. S., & Khan, R. N. 2020. Commentary on a combined approach to the problem of developing biomarkers for the prediction of spontaneous preterm labor that leads to preterm birth. *Placenta*, *98*, 13–23.

Lefkou, E., Mamopoulos, A., & Dagklis, T., *et al*. 2016. Pravastatin improves pregnancy outcomes in obstetric antiphospholipid syndrome refractory to antithrombotic therapy. *Journal of Clinical Investigation*, *126*, 2933–2940. 2016/07/28. DOI: 10.1172/jci86957.

Leow, S. M., Di Quinzio, M. K., Ng, Z. L., Grant, C., Amitay, T., Wei, Y., Hod, M., Sheehan, P. M., Brennecke, S. P., Arbel, N., & Georgiou, H. M. 2020. Preterm birth prediction in asymptomatic women at mid-gestation using a panel of novel protein biomarkers: The prediction of PreTerm Labor (PPeTaL) study. *American Journal of Obstetrics & Gynecology MFM*, *2*(2), 100084. https://doi.org/10.1159/000314018

Lev-Sagie, A., Goldman-Wohl, D., Cohen, Y., Dori-Bachash, M., Leshem, A., Mor, U., Strahilevitz, J., Moses, A. E., Shapiro, H., Yagel, S., & Elinav, E. 2019. Vaginal microbiome transplantation in women with intractable bacterial vaginosis. *Nature Medicine*, *25*(10), 1500–1504. https://doi.org/10.1159/000314018

Medley, N., Vogel, J. P., Care, A., & Alfirevic, Z., 2018. Interventions during pregnancy to prevent preterm birth: An overview of Cochrane systematic reviews. *Cochrane Database of Systematic Reviews*, (11).

Ozdemir, B. A., Karthikesalingam, A., Sinha, S., Poloniecki, J. D., Hinchliffe, R. J., Thompson, M. M., Gower, J. D., Boaz, A., & Holt, P. J. 2015. Research activity and the association with mortality. *PloS One*, *10*(2), e0118253. https://doi.org/10.1159/000314018

Petrou, L., Latvanen, E., Seichepine, F., Kim, S. H., Bennett, P. R., Sykes, L., MacIntyre, D. A., Terzidou, V., & Ladame, S. 2022. Lateral flow test (LFT) detects cell-free MicroRNAs predictive of preterm birth directly from human plasma. *Advanced NanoBiomed Research*, *2*(9), 2200026. https://doi.org/10.1159/000314018

Rosenbloom, J. I., Raghuraman, N., Temming, L. A., Stout, M. J., Tuuli, M. G., Dicke, J. M., Macones, G. A., & Cahill, A. G. 2020. Predictive value of midtrimester universal cervical length screening based on parity. *Journal of Ultrasound in Medicine*, *39*(1), 147–154. https://doi.org/10.1159/000314018

Sapantzoglou, I., Pergialiotis, V., Prokopakis, I., Douligeris, A., Stavros, S., Panagopoulos, P., Theodora, M., Antsaklis, P., & Daskalakis, G., 2023. Antibiotic therapy in patients with amniotic fluid sludge and risk of preterm birth: A meta-analysis. *Archives of Gynecology and Obstetrics*, *309*, 347–361.

Sheikh, A., Anderson, M., Albala, S., Casadei, B., Franklin, B. D., Richards, M., Taylor, D., Tibble, H., & Mossialos, E. 2021. Health information technology and digital innovation for national learning health and care systems. *The Lancet Digital Health*, *3*(6), e383–e396. https://doi.org/10.1159/000314018

Stewart, L. A., Simmonds, M., Duley, L., Llewellyn, A., Sharif, S., Walker, R. A., Beresford, L., Wright, K., Aboulghar, M. M., Alfirevic, Z., & Azargoon, A. 2021. Evaluating progestogens for preventing preterm birth international collaborative (EPPPIC): Meta-analysis of individual participant data from randomised controlled trials. *The Lancet, 397*(10280), 1183–1194. https://doi.org/10.1159/000314018

Surendiran, R., Aarthi, R., Thangamani, M., Sugavanam, S., & Sarumathy, R. 2022. A systematic review using machine learning algorithms for predicting preterm birth. *International Journal of Engineering Trends and Technology, 70*(5), 46–59. https://doi.org/10.1159/000314018

Vakili, S., Torabinavid, P., Tabrizi, R., Shojazadeh, A., Asadi, N., & Hessami, K., 2021. The association of inflammatory biomarker of neutrophil-to-lymphocyte ratio with spontaneous preterm delivery: A systematic review and meta-analysis. *Mediators of Inflammation, 2021*.

Vidal, M. S. Jr, Lintao, R. C., Severino, M. E. L., Tantengco, O. A. G., & Menon, R. 2022. Spontaneous preterm birth: Involvement of multiple feto-maternal tissues and organ systems, differing mechanisms, and pathways. *Frontiers in Endocrinology, 13*, 1015622.

Vieira-Baptista, P., De Seta, F., Verstraelen, H., Ventolini, G., Lonnee-Hoffmann, R., & Lev-Sagie, A. 2022. The vaginal microbiome: V. Therapeutic modalities of vaginal microbiome engineering and research challenges. *Journal of Lower Genital Tract Disease, 26*(1), 99. https://doi.org/10.1159/000314018

Wadon, M., Modi, N., Wong, H. S., Thapar, A., & O'Donovan, M. C. 2020. Recent advances in the genetics of preterm birth. *Annals of Human Genetics, 84*(3), 205–213. https://doi.org/10.1159/000314018

Zhang, Y., Lu, S., Wu, Y., Hu, W., & Yuan, Z. 2022. The prediction of preterm birth using time-series technology-based machine learning: Retrospective cohort study. *JMIR Medical Informatics, 10*(6), e33835. https://doi.org/10.1159/000314018

Appendix
Organisations providing support and information

BIRTH TRAUMA ASSOCIATION	**Birth Trauma Association:** supports women who have suffered a traumatic birth. The association does this by informing women that their feelings and experiences are validated. This is done through interactions with health professionals. **email:** enquiries@birthtraumaassociation.org.uk **Website: www.birthtraumaassociation.org**
Bliss for babies born premature or sick	**Bliss:** Charity for babies born premature or sick. They offer support and advice for parents and healthcare professionals. **Video Helpline** **https://www.bliss.org.uk/** **support-via-video-call-form** **Website: https://www.bliss.org.uk/**
The Lily Mae Foundation ® Supporting Parents & Families after a Stillbirth, Neonatal Death, Miscarriage or Medical Termination	**Lily Mae Foundation:** offers free advice and support to parents and families after a stillbirth or neonatal death. **Telephone: 01676 535 716** **Website: https://www.lilymaefoundation.org/**
Little heartbeats	**Little Heartbeats:** provides support and information to women who have experienced preterm prelabour rupture of membranes. **email:** little.heartbeats@mail.com **Website: https://www.little-heartbeats.org.uk/**
the lullaby trust safer sleep for babies ~ support for families	**The Lullaby Trust:** raises awareness of Sudden Infant Death Syndrome [SIDS] and offers free emotional support to bereaved families. **Telephone: 0808 802 6868** **Website: https://www.lullabytrust.org.uk/**

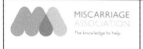	**Miscarriage Association:** provides support to those who have experienced a miscarriage, ectopic, or molar pregnancy. **Telephone:** 01924 200 799 **Website: https://www.miscarriageassociation.org.uk/**
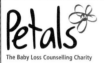	**Petals: Baby Loss Counselling Charity:** provides specialist counselling after baby loss. **Telephone:** 0300 688 0068 **Email:** counselling@petalscharity.org **Website: https://petalscharity.org/**
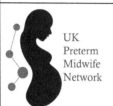	**Preterm Birth Specialist Midwives Group:** a network of midwives working in the field of preterm birth who share questions, advice and new developments in the field. **To join the network please visit:** www.networks.nhs.uk and search "preterm"
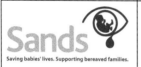	**SANDS:** is a charity working to save babies' lives and support bereaved families through its Freephone helpline, online community and resources, and around 110 regional support groups. They also support research and provide training for health care professionals (contact:training@sands.org.uk). **Telephone:** 0808 164 3332 **Website: https://www.sands.org.uk/**
Tommy's The pregnancy and baby charity	**Tommy's, the pregnancy and baby charity:** Provides evidence-based health information before, during and after pregnancy to parents to help them have a healthy baby. Provides the My Prem Baby app for parents of premature babies. Has a midwife-led helpline and a special helpline for Black and Black Mixed-Heritage women to discuss any aspect of pregnancy, premature birth or pregnancy loss. Invests £2m annually into research to prevent preterm birth, miscarriage and stillbirth. **Telephone:** 0800 0147 800 **Website: https://www.tommys.org/**
	UK Preterm Clinical Network: is a network of doctors, midwives and scientists committed to improving preterm birth care and outcomes. **To be added to the email mailing list please email:** jenny.carter@kcl.ac.uk or ukpcn@kcl.ac.uk

Index